Jean-Luc Wautier
Marie-Paule Wautier

Molecular mechanism of erythrocyte adhesion to endothelium

Jean-Luc Wautier
Marie-Paule Wautier

Molecular mechanism of erythrocyte adhesion to endothelium

Overview and advances

LAP LAMBERT Academic Publishing

Impressum / Imprint

Bibliografische Information der Deutschen Nationalbibliothek: Die Deutsche Nationalbibliothek verzeichnet diese Publikation in der Deutschen Nationalbibliografie; detaillierte bibliografische Daten sind im Internet über http://dnb.d-nb.de abrufbar.
Alle in diesem Buch genannten Marken und Produktnamen unterliegen warenzeichen-, marken- oder patentrechtlichem Schutz bzw. sind Warenzeichen oder eingetragene Warenzeichen der jeweiligen Inhaber. Die Wiedergabe von Marken, Produktnamen, Gebrauchsnamen, Handelsnamen, Warenbezeichnungen u.s.w. in diesem Werk berechtigt auch ohne besondere Kennzeichnung nicht zu der Annahme, dass solche Namen im Sinne der Warenzeichen- und Markenschutzgesetzgebung als frei zu betrachten wären und daher von jedermann benutzt werden dürften.

Bibliographic information published by the Deutsche Nationalbibliothek: The Deutsche Nationalbibliothek lists this publication in the Deutsche Nationalbibliografie; detailed bibliographic data are available in the Internet at http://dnb.d-nb.de.
Any brand names and product names mentioned in this book are subject to trademark, brand or patent protection and are trademarks or registered trademarks of their respective holders. The use of brand names, product names, common names, trade names, product descriptions etc. even without a particular marking in this works is in no way to be construed to mean that such names may be regarded as unrestricted in respect of trademark and brand protection legislation and could thus be used by anyone.

Coverbild / Cover image: www.ingimage.com

Verlag / Publisher:
LAP LAMBERT Academic Publishing
ist ein Imprint der / is a trademark of
AV Akademikerverlag GmbH & Co. KG
Heinrich-Böcking-Str. 6-8, 66121 Saarbrücken, Deutschland / Germany
Email: info@lap-publishing.com

Herstellung: siehe letzte Seite /
Printed at: see last page
ISBN: 978-3-659-24441-4

Copyright © 2013 AV Akademikerverlag GmbH & Co. KG
Alle Rechte vorbehalten. / All rights reserved. Saarbrücken 2013

Table of Contents

Introduction	page 3
Sickle Cell Disease	page 5
Gaucher disease	page 13
Malaria	page 16
Diabetes mellitus	page 21
Polycythemia Vera	page 31
Retinal Vein Occlusion	page 39
Conclusion	page 46
References	page 48

Introduction

Since the battle between Virchow (German) and Cruveiller (French) during the 19th century about the origin of vessel inflammation few progresses have been made since the 20th century. This was an European controversy forgotten. The work of W. Osler, in England than in Canada, who discovered that inflammation was a main factor in vessel dysfunction.

After the lipid origin of atherosclerosis new evidence showed that lipids were important and most of them are oxidized lipids stimulating an inflammatory reaction at the vessel site. Beside the anatomic observation, experimental research demonstrated that several factors were involved in atherosclerosis: Infection disease, metabolic disorders, leading in vascular alterations initiating atherothrombosis. Several improvements were made first: Lipid metabolism correction, better diabetes control achieved, antithrombotic drugs improved but at least the war was not won and investigations were needed.

In this chapter we try to demonstrate that unknown factors are responsible for vascular dysfunction and can be countered by new therapeutical approaches.

Endothelium was considered as a non-reactive surface however when endothelial cell culture was possible, the physiology of endothelium was explored.

The interactions between blood cells, including leukocytes red blood cells and platelets, and vessels are essential in inflammatory situations, infectious and thrombotic diseases. During the last two decades numerous researches have been conducted to identify molecular and physical parameters involved in these phenomena. It is more recently that has been recognized the importance of red cell adhesion to endothelium in the occurrence of thrombotic complications. We were pioneers in this field of research and have chosen for this development six examples in which the molecular basis has been well identified. Biochemical analysis of membrane components, sequencing of proteins and glycoproteins have allowed discover that they belonged to families of molecules whose function was already discovered in cell/cell interactions.

Sickle Cell Disease (SCD)

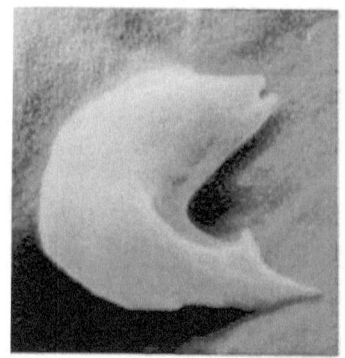 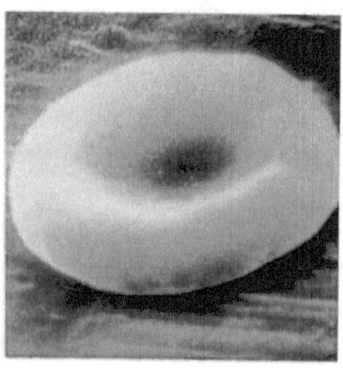

Sickle Red Blood Cell **Normal Red Blood Cell**

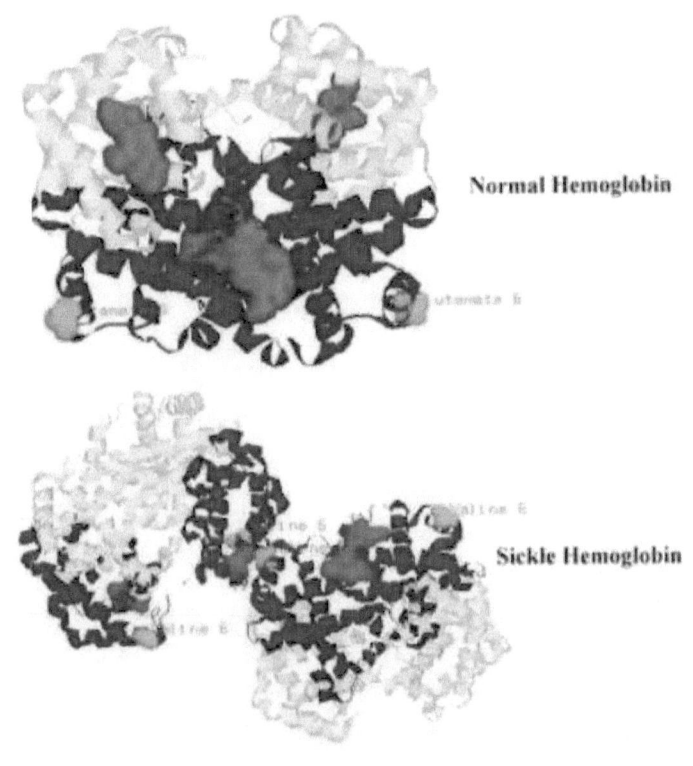

6

Hemoglobin A: βchain Val-His-Leu-Thr-Pro-**Glu**-Glu-Lys......

Hemoglobin S: βchain Val-His-Leu-Thr-Pro-**Val**-Glu-Lys......

Note: The Sickle hemoglobin image is drawn at 50% of the size of the normal hemoglobin

Sickle Cell Disease (SCD)

Sickle cell disease is secondary to a mutation of hemoglobin and the patients have either hemoglobin S (HbSS) or are heterozygous (HbSC). Sickle cell disease was the first disease in which abnormalities of RBC structure could be associated with functional abnormalities. The sickling observed when the oxygen partial pressure is reduced is the consequence of hemoglobin S polymerization, is accompanied by reduced deformability of red blood cells. It was a first possible explanation for the phenomena of vascular occlusion observed at high altitude and during air travel. However, individuals with sickle cell disease, homozygous (HbSS) or double heterozygous (HbSC), have vascular occlusions outside period of oxygen deprivation. Another pathophysiological mechanism has to be found. R. Hebbel [1] was the first to demonstrate that red blood cells from sickle cell patients have a pathological adherence to the vascular endothelium. It is through the culture of endothelial cells and the use of red blood cells labeled with 51 Chromium that it was possible to demonstrate an increased adhesion of red blood cells of sickle cell patients. We have shown that adherence is greater when blood is taken when patients have vaso-occlusive episodes [2]. Moreover this phenomenon is enhanced by proteins such as fibrinogen [3]. The protein associated with blood group Lutheran Lu/BCAM, when the protein kinase A is activated, is phosphorylated [4]. This phosphorylation significantly increases its affinity for laminin, a protein found in the subendothelium but also expressed on the apical endothelial cell [5], this largely explains the excessive red blood cell adhesion. Reticulocytes express at a relatively high level a molecule already known for leukocyte adhesive properties, VLA-4 (integrin α4β1). Counterpart of the molecule VLA-4 is Vascular Cell Adhesion Molecule 1 (VCAM-1).

The pathophysiology of SCD is complex and not fully understood. RBC adhesion to the vascular wall probably favors the formation of HbS polymers by slowing the flow of cells circulating through capillaries, thereby leading to the next step, which is vaso-occlusion. Several observations support the hypothesis that abnormal cell adhesion plays an important role in the obstruction of microvessels or in facilitating the trapping of sickle cells in postcapillary venules. In SCD patients, transit of red blood cells (RBCs) into small vessels could be slowed by their abnormal adhesion to the vascular wall through interactions between erythroid adhesion molecules and proteins on the surface of endothelial cells or extracellular matrix (ECM) components. Several interactions have been described between SS RBCs and the endothelial vascular wall. Integrin VLA-4 expressed on young circulating reticulocytes, is a major actor in these interactions through its binding to VCAM-1, fibronectin, thrombospondin (TSP) and endothelial Lutheran/basal cell-adhesion molecule (Lu/BCAM) to laminin [6]. TSP mediates adhesion of SS reticulocytes to endothelial cells by bridging CD36 molecules expressed on both cell types [7]. However, the clinical severity of SCD in CD36-deficient patients is not diminished [8]. Landsteiner–Weiner/intercellular adhesion molecule-4 (LW/ICAM-4) and Lu/BCAM are members of the immunoglobulin superfamily, expressed on young and mature RBCs; they are also involved in the abnormal adhesion of SS RBCs through interactions with endothelial integrin αVβ3 and ECM laminin 511/521, respectively [9]. Sickle-cell disease is characterized by painful episodic vaso-occlusive crises (VOC), acute chest syndrome and a chronic inflammatory state. Hydroxyurea (HU) is the only drug now available having demonstrated benefit for SCD patients, with fewer VOC and acute chest syndromes [10], and lower mortality and morbidity. HU diminishes SS RBC adhesion to endothelial cells and the ECM proteins, fibronectin, TSP and laminin. These decreases are consistent with less CD36, $\alpha 4\beta 1$ and LW/ICAM-4 expression on the surface of SS reticulocytes and erythrocytes.

Peptides (Synthetic peptides FWV and ATSR comprising amino acids on the A and G, strands of ICAM-4 domain 1, respectively) based on αV-binding domains of ICAM-4 on sickle erythrocytes bind to endothelial cells via $\alpha V\beta 3$ and this interaction can significantly contribute to vaso-occlusion in sickle cell disease. In the ex-vivo mesoceum preparation infusion of synthetic peptides markedly improved hemodynamic behavior of sickle erythrocytes. In preparations in which Platelet Activating Factor (PAF) treatment was followed by incubation with αV-binding peptide FWV or ATSR, infusion of sickle erythrocytes resulted in significant decreases in peripheral vascular resistance compared with preparations treated with PAF alone. In marked contrast, treatment with a control peptide had no effect. In preparations treated with PAF alone, adhesion of sickle erythrocytes showed a strong inverse correlation with venular diameter, which is in agreement with published observations. Neither FWV nor ATSR caused blockage in postcapillary venules, in marked contrast to the extensive blockage observed after infusion of sickle erythrocytes in preparations treated with PAF alone [11].

In both human with sickle cell disease and transgenic sickle mice, chronic inflammatory activation of endothelium results in upregulation of endothelial adhesion molecules (i.e., VCAM-1, ICAM-1, E-selectin, P-selectin, and $\alpha V\beta 3$-

integrin). However, the mechanistic aspects of red blood cell adhesion in transgenic sickle mice are not fully understood, and the substances that stimulate or inhibit red cell adhesion in transgenic mice are yet to be characterized. In contrast, the ex vivo model used, similar to cultured human endothelial cells, allows testing known stimulating and inhibitory agents on adhesion of human SS red blood cells. Importantly, the ex vivo model allows distinction of microvascular sites and characteristics of adhesion and vaso-occlusion under conditions of shear flow. Thus the use of the ex vivo preparation is relevant to identify the ICAM-4 domains involved in human SS red blood cell adhesion in the microcirculation. It would be important in future studies to validate these findings in relevant sickle mouse models, as well as establish the contribution of plasma factors and other blood cells to ICAM-4-mediated sickle vaso-occlusion.

It was shown that ICAM-4 is unique among the ICAM family in that it interacts with multiple integrins, including $\alpha L\beta 2$ (LFA-1) and $\alpha M\beta 2$ (Mac-1) on leukocytes, the fibrinogen receptor $\alpha IIb\beta 3$ (GpIIb/IIIa) on platelets, as well as $\alpha 4\beta 1$- and αV-integrins. Thus ICAM-4 has multiple domains that bind diverse integrins, some of which may have important roles in cell-cell interactions in sickle cell disease. Hence, the possibility exists that ICAM-4 may be involved in various dynamic cell-cell interactions during vaso-occlusion, including sickle red cells with endothelial cells, neutrophils, and platelets. The spatial relationship of integrin binding sites on the surface of ICAM-4 is emerging. Interestingly, the area on ICAM-4 important for its interaction with αV-integrins is adjacent to, but distinct from, the binding sites previously identified for the ICAM-4-binding partners $\alpha L\beta 2$ and $\alpha M\beta 2$.

Hydroxyurea (HU), also called hydroxycarbamide, is the only drug now available having demonstrated benefit for SCD patients. It was commonly thought that HU acted as an antisickling agent by increasing fetal hemoglobin

(HbF) levels, leading to significantly less hemoglobin S polymerization. Lu/BCAM, the unique erythroid receptors of laminin, a major ECM protein, is expressed in young and mature RBC, unlike CD36 and integrin $\alpha_4\beta_1$, which are restricted to reticulocytes.

HU significantly increased erythroid Lu/BCAM expression by enhancing both the percentage of Lu/BCAM-positive RBC and the numbers of Lu/BCAM copies/RBC. Hydroxyurea did not modulate the alternative splicing generating Lu and Lu(v13) isoforms but rather up-regulated erythroid expression of the Lu gene. As expected, HU increased the Hb concentration and HbF percentage. The reduced RBC adhesion to laminin under HU was associated to a decreased Lu/BCAM long isoform phosphorylation (Bartolucci P Blood 2010) despite its enhanced expression. This decreased phosphorylation was most probably a direct consequence of the diminished intracellular cAMP levels measured in these patients during HU treatment. As intracellular cAMP levels are controlled by several effectors including adenylyl cyclase and phosphodiesterases, further studies are needed to fully characterize the HU mechanism of action in SCD. Some observations suggested that HU might raise nitric oxide levels by stimulating vascular endothelial cell production of it *via* the eNOS–cGMP pathway. HU could also prevent neutrophil activation and adhesion to fibronectin in a cAMP–PKA-dependent manner. The *in vivo* effect of HU on Lu/BCAM long isoform phosphorylation and cAMP decrease could not be tested *ex vivo* using SS RBCs because of hemolysis. Using human erythroleukemic K562-Lu cells expressing recombinant Lu gp, it was shown that the *ex vivo* effects of HU were similar to those observed for SS RBCs from HU-treated SCD patients. [12].

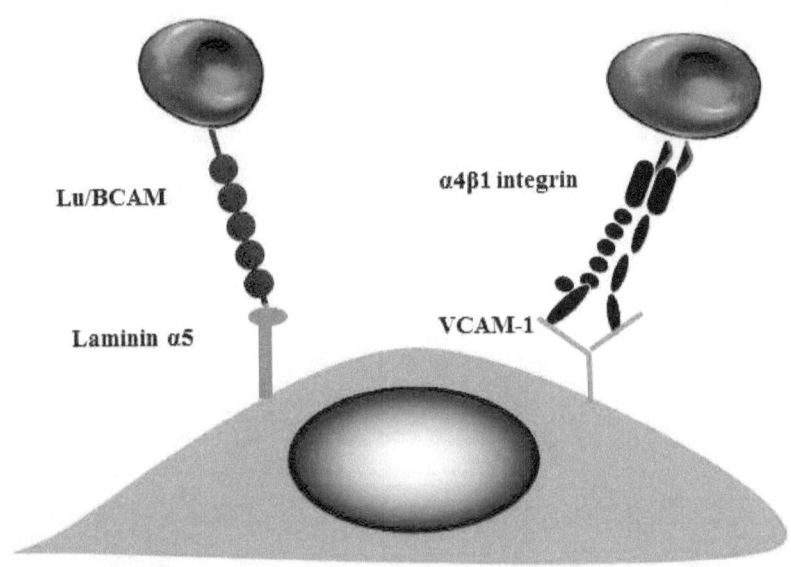

Sickle Cell Disease

The protein associated with blood group Lutheran Lu/BCAM binds to Lamininin α5, a protein found in the subendothelium but also expressed on the apical endothelial cell. Reticulocytes express at a relatively high level a molecule already known for its adhesive properties of leukocytes; it is VLA-4 (integrin α4β1). Counterpart of the molecule VLA-4 is Vascular Cell Adhesion Molecule-1 (VCAM-1)

Gaucher disease

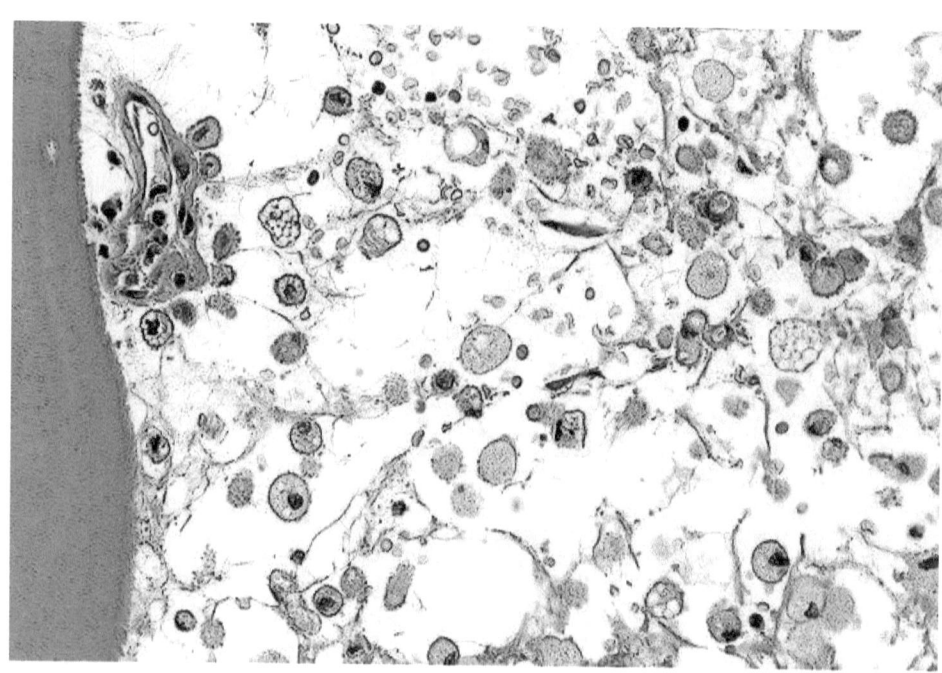

Micrograph showing crinkled paper macrophages in the marrow space in a case of Gaucher disease. H&E stain.

Gaucher disease

Gaucher disease (GD) is caused by β-glucocerebrosidase (GluCerase) deficiency. GD is a multisystem disorder with high clinical heterogeneity. Ten percent of GD patients, including fetuses (fetal GD), infants (type2), older children and adults (type 3) have signs of central nervous system involvement. However the majority of patients belong to the subgroup of nonneuronopathic GD (type 1).

GluCerase deficiency results in the accumulation of glucosylceramide (GlcCer) into macrophages. GlcCer-laden macrophages are not killed by the accumulation of the substrate, but tend to transform into Gaucher cells.

In vitro studies and animal models showed that GluCerase deficiency reduced the differentiation of bone marrow stem cells into osteoblasts [13; 14], and alters the proliferation and differenciation capacity of CD34+cells [15]. Thus, it appears that the complex pathophysiology of GD may involve a wide array of cell types and processes.

Red Blood Cells (RBC) on Giemsa stained peripheral blood smears exhibited significantly greater proportion of abnormal RBC shapes in GD patients compared with normal samples. Dacryocytes ("tear drop" cells), elliptocytes, echinocytes and shistocytes were observed. GD RBC deformability was reduced compared with normal RBC. Hemorheologic data suggest membrane alterations in GD RBCand may explain the abnormal RBC shape in GD. Significant proportion of RBC from GD patients with an intact spleen and not under enzyme replacement therapy have abnormal shapes.

GD has been considered as a primarily macrophage-specific glucosphingolidosis but recent studies demonstrated the involvement of erythroid cells in GD pathophysiology.

The adhesion to endothelial cells and to laminin of GD RBC was significantly higher compared to that of normal RBC. Lu/BCAM is overexpressed and highly phosphorylated in GD RBC [16]. Increased RBC adhesion may be related to the accumulation of GlcCer into RBC membranes and the abnormal lipid membrane composition resulting in Lu/BCAM activation.

Malaria

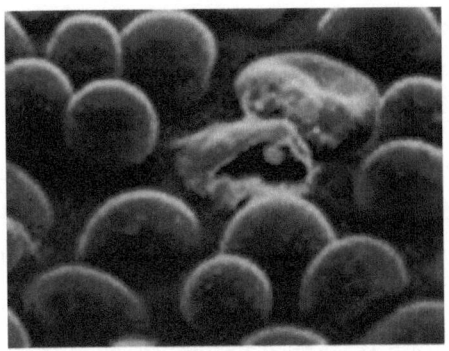

Microscopic magnification shows *Plasmodium falciparum*, the most virulent of the four malaria parasites.

Photograph by Albert Bonniers Forlag

Malaria

Plasmodium Falciparum is responsible for more than one million deaths per year affecting mainly children in Africa [17] but is also an important public health problem in South East Asia [18]. The consequence of sequestration of red cells in the microcirculation is an important element of the pathophysiology. The adhesion to endothelium is mediated by a parasite protein, *plasmodium falciparum* erythrocyte membrane protein 1 (PfEMP1). Its pathogenesis is closely associated with the adhesive properties of the variable erythrocyte surface antigens, PfEMP1, encoded by the *var* gene family [19]. Based on distinct types of promoter sequences and their internal versus telomeric chromosomal location, the 60 member *var* gene family of the sequenced 3D7 clone can be classified into related groups. There are three major groups, (A, B, and C), two intermediate groups (B/A and B/C) and the more distantly related *var1* and *var2csa* genes. Mutation and recombination have generated a vast repertoire of polymorphic variants and how this antigenic variation system operates during infection is a major question in malaria biology and clinical research [20]. The complete *plasmodium falciparum* 3D7 genome sequence and real-time quantitative RT-PCR enable accurate measurement of the relative amounts of *var* gene transcripts in intra-erythrocytic malaria parasite populations. *Plasmodium falciparum* erythrocyte membrane protein 1 is a large molecule consisting of regions similar to the outer region of Duffy. Inter Cellular Adhesion Molecule-1 (ICAM-1) is involved in cerebral malaria and appears as a ligand for PfEMP1 [21]. CD36 is present on the endothelium and weakly expressed in the brain. It could be involved in the adhesion of red blood cells infected by the parasite. Other structures such as endothelial CD31 and glycosaminoglycans also bind to PfEMP1 [17] PfEMP1 proteins have multiple domains and most CIDR-α type domains bind CD36 [22] while some DBLβc2 domains bind ICAM-1 and some single PfEMP1 species have been shown to mediate multiple independent interactions with a diverse set of host receptors including CD31/PECAM-1, the blood group A antigen, normal nonimmune IgM, heparan sulfate–like glucosaminoglycan, and CD36 [23]. The red blood cell interaction with endothelium is complex, variable depending on the location of the endothelium. A study has suggested that the ability of parasites to bind to multiple receptors is correlated with disease severity. In addition, several lines of evidence have implicated CD54/ICAM-1, CD31/PECAM-1 [24] as well as PFD1235w and PF11_0008 as having a role in severe disease. A potential mechanism for the two PfEMP1 interactions could involve a role for PFD1235w as a primary ligand for rolling and CD54/ICAM-1 binding on the endothelium thus enabling further contacts with CD31/PECAM-1 which could be mediated by PF11_0008, when both are present on the infected erythrocyte surface.

Plasmodium falciparum Antigen 332 (Pf332) is the largest parasite protein (approx. 700 kDa) that is exported into the infected-parasite red blood cell cytosol. Pf332 is synthesized by the intracellular malaria parasite and exported to the RBC via Maurer's clefts (MC) where it associates with the RBC membrane skeleton. The current membrane topology of Pf332 predicts that the N-terminal 540 residue region of Pf332 (encoded by exon 1) is located in either in the lumen of an organelle (the MC) or extracellularly exposed on the RBC. This prediction seems reasonable as this domain contains a Duffy Binding-Like (DBL) domain which is rich in cysteine residues that are likely to form numerous disulphide bonds, which can only occur in an oxidizing environment found inside trafficking organelles or extracellularly. Therefore, the sequences encoded by exon one of *pf332* would not be present within the same biological compartment as the RBC membrane skeleton [25].

The recent identification of a group of novel protein kinases (serine/Threonine protein kinase , FIKK family) within the Plasmodium falciparum genome has provided researchers with a basis for what many hope to be new potential drug targets for malaria.

In the human malaria parasite Plasmodium falciparum, potential candidates for erythrocyte remodelling include the apicomplexan-specific FIKK kinase family (20 members), several of which have been demonstrated to be transported into the erythrocyte cytoplasm via Maurer's clefts. Two members of the FIKK kinase family are involved in the remodeling of erythrocyte membrane skeleton proteins. Importantly, each analyzed FIKK member apparently targets a distinct protein at a different time point of the asexual blood cycle. Recent studies [26] suggest that FIKK12 targets a protein of 80 kDa at trophozoite stage and FIKK7.1 targets another protein of approx. 300 kDa at schizont stage. A recent study reported changes in the phosphoproteome of IEs and identified numerous *P. falciparum* phosphorylated proteins and 77 human proteins as phosphorylated in IEs whereas only 48 were detected in uninfected erythrocytes. This indicates an elevated level of post-translational modifications of the host cell by parasite kinases. Given that most of the *Pf fikk* genes were shown to be transcribed in blood stages and N-terminal regions are unique to each paralog, this raises the possibility that each FIKK protein might have different functions in the IEs and that other FIKK proteins could have other biological roles including trafficking, adhesion and antigenic variation.

Adhesion would then be improved through simultaneous binding to several receptors [27].The expression of endothelial adhesion molecules can be modulated by cytokines such as TNF - alpha or TGF - beta. The treatment of malaria also interferes with the production of PfEMP1 and thus have an effect on the phenomenon of adhesion.

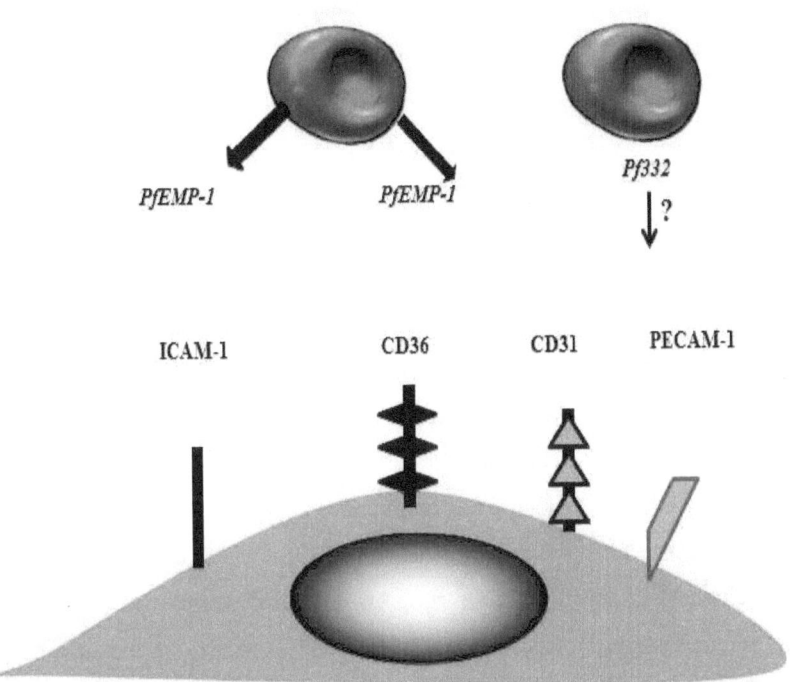

Malaria

The red blood cell interaction with endothelium is complex, variable depending on the location of the endothelium. Inter Cellular Adhesion Molecule (ICAM-1) appears as a ligand for *Plasmodium falciparum* erythrocyte membrane protein1 (PfEMP1). CD36 present on the endothelium could be involved in the adhesion of red blood cells infected by the parasite. Other structures such as endothelial CD31, Platelet Endothelial Cell Adhesion Molecule-1 (PECAM-1) and glycosaminoglycans also bind to PfEMP1.

Diabetes mellitus

Since diabetes was defined by Claude Bernard we know that it is a major risk factor for vascular thrombosis. The increase in blood glucose is often associated with lipid disorders and platelet hyperactivity. Premature cardiovascular disease is the most common cause of morbidity and mortality, but the microvascular complications specific to diabetes are also contributory factors. Diabetes is the most frequent cause for renal replacement therapy. It is also the most common cause of blindness in developed countries. About half of patients with diabetes develop microalbuminuria. Approximately 30% will progress to proteinuria and 50% to renal failure. In UKPDS, tight control of blood pressure (144/82 *v* 154/87 mm Hg) reduced the incidence of a microvascular event by 37%. A 13% reduction in risk for microvascular event can be achieved with the reduction in systolic blood pressure of 10 mm Hg. In addition, angiotensin converting enzyme inhibitors prevent microalbuminuria and nephropathy with the best accuracy [28; 29; 30; 31]

Diabetes provides a model of chronic vascular disease in which disordered glucose homeostasis triggers abnormalities eventuating in dysfunction of virtually every organ, deriving, in part, from vascular perturbation. Although superimposition of other risk factors, such as hyperlipemia or hypertension, adds to the complex atherogenic milieu, diabetes by itself is a well-recognized independent cardiovascular risk factor [32; 33; 34; 35; 36].

Non-enzymatic glycosylation of proteins results in the formation of advanced glycation end products (AGE: Carboxymethyl-lysine CML, Methylglyoxal MG), which are considered as toxic factors damaging vessels. In 1981 we have been able to demonstrate, using the same system as that described by Hebbel that red cells of diabetic patients have increased adhesion to endothelium and the adhesion is correlated with the severity of vascular injury [37]. We have, in a group of diabetic patients followed for one year, observed that in the same patient adherence intensity evolved in parallel with glycated hemoglobin HbA1c [38].

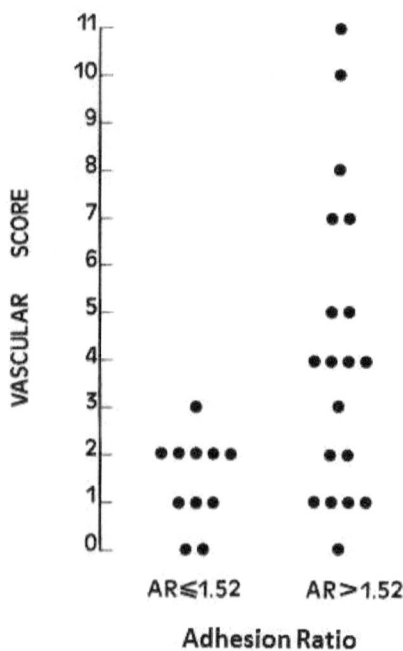

The mean adhesion ratio (percentage of adhering diabetic red cells/percentage of adhering control red cells) was 2.33 (range, 0.8 to 5.2). Increased adhesion was related to the extent of vascular complications in the diabetics, as assessed by a vascular score.

Thirteen years later we discovered the molecular basis responsible for adhesion [39]. The adhesion of diabetic erythrocytes to endothelium is mediated by a specific interaction between AGE present on erythrocyte and a specific receptor (RAGE) on endothelium.

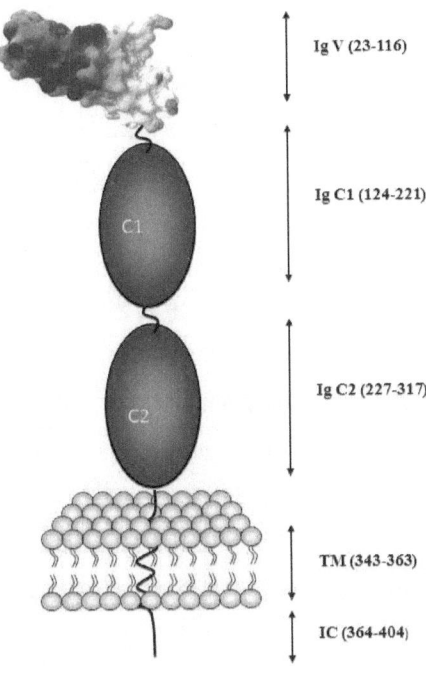

RAGE is a member of the immunoglobulin (Ig) superfamily that contains three Ig-like domains, one variable (V) and two constant (C1 and C2), in the extracellular part, a single transmembrane domain (TM) and one short cytosolic tail.

Consistant with this hypothesis was the observation that infusion of diabetic red blood cells (RBC) into normal rats resulted in an accelerated clearance, which was blocked in large part by anti-RAGE IgG [39]. These data suggest that diabetic RBCs exhibit enhanced interaction with RAGE expressed by the blood vessels in vivo. The major significance could be the induction of oxidant stress, which was observed in vitro and in vivo after erythrocyte-endothelium interaction. The consequence of the interaction between diabetic RBC and endothelium results in several perturbations such as an increased permeability and a potentiation in interleukin-6 (IL-6) production. The oxidant stress secondary to RBC adhesion induces the activation of $NF_\kappa B$. The effect can be prevented by the addition of antioxidant such as probucol suggesting that the production of reactive oxygen intermediates is involved in the cellular transmission mechanism. The presence of RAGE in different cell types suggests that it could be involved in the genesis of diabetic complications but the exact implication of AGE-RAGE interaction need additional evidences such as the effect of receptor blockade on end organ damage. Other therapeutical approaches using iloprost or sulprostone inhibits the adhesion of diabetic RBC to endothelium as well as cell permeability or IL-6 production [40]. The partial or total correction of the endothelial cell perturbations provoked by the adhesion of diabetic erythrocytes suggest that the effect of iloprost could be due to an action on the intracellular endothelial cell function.

RAGE engagement by ligands activates multiple signalling pathways including p21ras, ERK1/2 (p44/p42), p38 MAPkinase, SAPK/JNK MAPkinases, rho GTPases, phosphoinositol-3 kinase and the JAK/STAT pathway, and downstream effectors such as $NF\kappa B$ and CREB [41]. Engagement of RAGE by AGE triggers the generation of reactive oxygen species (ROS). The incubation of human endothelial cells with Carboxymethyl-Lysine (CML), present on plasma proteins or RBC membrane proteins, prompted intracellular generation of hydrogen peroxide, a process suppressed by diphenyliodonium (DPI) but not by inhibitors of nitric oxide (NO). DPI may inhibit other flavoprotein dehydrogenases in addition to NADPH oxidase. Macrophages derived from wild-type mice exhibit enhanced levels of tissue factor (TF) on stimulation with AGE, corroborating the important role for NADPH oxidase in AGE–RAGE–triggered events. On the contrary, macrophages derived from gp91phox deficient mice failed to display enhanced TF expression on incubation with AGEs [42]. Forearm resistance vessel responses to endothelium dependent and independent agonists are abnormal in individuals with type 1 diabetes. Patients with the highest HbA1c levels showed the most marked impairment in the response to acetylcholine. This is consistent with either reduced vascular smooth muscle cell responsiveness to NO or NO bioavailability. Increased vascular permeability is characteristic of early diabetic vasculopathy. Post confluent cultured endothelial cells incubated with red blood cells from diabetic patients revealed increased diffusional transit (permeability of macromolecular tracers ^{125}I-albumin and ^{3}H-inulin) compared with endothelial cells incubated with red blood cells from non-diabetic subjects. The diminution of endothelial cell barrier function was completely inhibited by anti-RAGE antibodies. Furthermore, the administration of recombinant soluble RAGE in diabetic rats, hyperpermeability was blocked in intestine and skin and suppressed by 90% in the kidney. Inhibition of AGE and diabetic hyperpermeability by antioxidants both in vitro and in vivo suggested a central role of AGE–RAGE–induced oxidant stress in the development of hyperpermeability [43; 44]. These studies strongly suggested that reactive oxygen species formation is a likely means by which oxidative stress can reversibly increase vascular permeability by rapid changes in endothelial cell shape via calcium mediated pathways. The quenching of NO by reactive oxygen species can also increase permeability [45]. The presence of micro vascular complications (retinopathy, nephropathy) is correlated with elevated serum levels of AGEs; both of these conditions are associated with increased vascular permeability [46]. Nitric Oxide (NO) formation inhibition by nitro-L-arginine potentiated RBC adhesion from diabetic patients to endothelium [47]. On the opposite, the addition of NO donors (NOR-3, SIN-1 or SNAP) reduced or inhibited adhesion of RBC from diabetic patients measured in flow conditions.

Activation of NADPH oxidase is a key process by which AGE, via RAGE, generates reactive oxygen species (ROS) and triggers signal transduction events that lead to altered gene expression in endothelial cells and macrophages. NADPH oxidase is a major source of ROS in vascular cells. Membrane subunit gp91phox and p22phox and the cytosolic subunit p67phox and p47phox and the small GTPase rac1 assemble and form the functional enzyme. DPI or HMAP, another inhibitor of NADPH oxidase, suppress AGE-mediated generation of ROS. NADPH oxidase is unregulated in spontaneously hypertensive rats and markers of oxidative stress are elevated in untreated rats [48]. The enhanced activity of tissue factor (TF) in AGE-stimulated macrophages harvested from gp91phox-null mice is suppressed compared with wild-type macrophages. This indicates the important role of NADPH oxidase in AGE-mediated processes. Importantly, recent studies indicating that endothelial cells express a gp91phox-containing NADPH oxidase support our hypothesis that activation of this enzyme provides a source of ROS upon AGE engagement of RAGE. In those studies by Gorlach et al. [49], it was shown that NADPH oxidase was a major source of ROS generation in the arterial wall, because its activation was associated with impaired bioavailability of endothelium-derived NO. Angiotensin II is a potent stimulus for ROS production in vascular cells, one of the main action is the activation of NADPH oxidase [50]. A strong correlation was found between vascular disease with reduced synthesis of NO and elevated levels of asymmetrical dimethylarginine (ADMA) suggesting that ADMA can be viewed as an endogenous inhibitor of NO synthase (NOS). ADMA, significantly increased in diabetic animals and in various cardiovascular and renal diseases, likely impair the modulation of arteriolar resistance by NO [51].

The reduction of endothelial RAGE expression by thiazolidinediole (TZDs) decreases the cell susceptibility toward AGE-related inflammation, as shown by impaired MCP-1 release after TZD pre-treatment. In contrast, TZDs did not affect TNF-α–induced MCP-1 expression, ruling out a direct effect of Peroxisome Proliferator Activator Receptor (PPAR-γ activators) [52]. These data might have important physiopathological and clinical implications for the high-risk population of diabetic patients: these patients do exhibit simultaneously increased AGE levels and enhanced RAGE expression in the vasculature. In vascular cells like endothelial cells, AGE-RAGE interaction leads to a long lasting and extensive expression of pro-atherogenic mediators, such as MCP-1 or VCAM-1. TNF-α, one of the cytokines released from these inflammatory cells in the plaque, may then in turn increase endothelial RAGE expression, thus creating a vicious circle that perpetuates the atherogenic process in diabetic patients. Data from animal experiments demonstrated that interruption of the AGE-RAGE interaction decreases lesion size in a mouse model of arteriosclerosis[53]. Limiting RAGE activation or RAGE expression by antidiabetic TZDs may be considered a therapeutic tool to influence vascular disease in diabetic patients.

In Diabetes Mellitus RBC Band 3 protein is glycated and binds to the receptor for Advanced Glycation End Products (RAGE) [54]. Protein glycation is associated with a high risk of vascular complications, especially in the microcirculation responsible for retinopathy and diabetic nephropathy [55]. Inhibition of AGE formation in animal models prevents or reduces the occurrence of vascular complications [56]. In human the most effective strategies are currently a good balance of diabetes treatment. Unfortunately anti free radical molecules such as vitamin E, is not effective at the doses which may be administered in humans. Modulation of expression of the receptor RAGE [57] or blocking its functions are potential new therapeutical approaches [58].

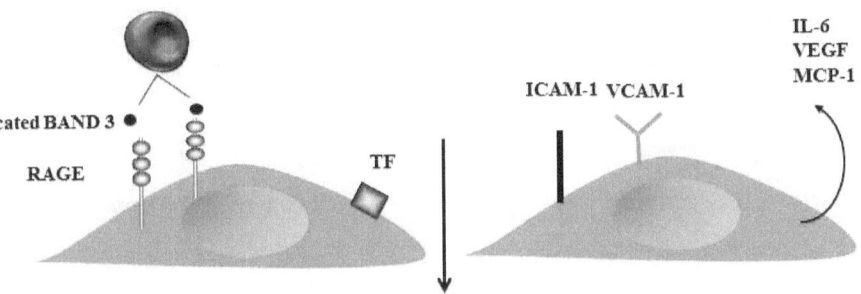

Diabetes mellitus

RBC Band 3 protein is glycated in patients with diabetes mellitus and binds to the receptor for Advanced Glycation End Products (RAGE). Engagement of endothelial RAGE induced Tissue Factor (TF) production, Intercellular Cell Adhesion Molecule-1 (ICAM-1) and Vascular Cell Adhesion Molecule (VCAM-1) expression, and IL-6, Vascular Endothelial Growth Factor (VEGF), Macrophage Chemoattractant Protein-1 (MCP-1) release. Diabetic red blood cells increased vascular permeability

Polycythemia Vera

Polycythemia vera (PV) is a chronic disorder in which the clonal proliferation of multipotent hematopoietic cells results in an increase in the red cell mass. This expansion is associated with circulatory disturbances mostly related to hyperviscosity. PV is the most common myeloproliferative syndrome [59], characterized by erythropoietin-independent erythroid colony formation *in vitro*, and was recently shown to be associated in most cases to a somatic point mutation of the JAK2 tyrosine kinase (JAK2 V617F) [60; 61; 62]. Since the first description of PV in 1892 in a patient with thrombosis, several criteria have been used to characterize this disorder: determination of red cell mass, the bone marrow culture, and more recently JAK2 mutation. Thrombotic complications are frequent in PV patients, and in particular cerebrovascular events. In the Budd-chiari syndrome, post-sinusoidal obstruction may occur outside the liver in the hepatic veins and this is frequently observed in patients with PV where no other thrombosis is detectable. The variability in the expression of adhesion molecules along the vascular tree and differences in flow conditions might explain why the occurrence of thrombosis is not at random. The number of patients investigated our study does not allow us to determine whether or not Lu/BCAM overexpression and/or phosphorylation is an index of thrombotic risk in PV patients, but JAK2 V617F mutation has been reported as a risk factor for thrombosis [63].

However the optimal management of patients with PV remains controversial. Phlebotomy and aspirin are still the first line therapy but despite the red cell mass reduction, the risk of thrombosis remains higher than in a population of sex and age matched subjects. In addition the use of anti-platelet agents can increase the risk of hemorrhage. Since adhesion of red blood cell (RBC) to endothelium was shown to be correlated to vascular risk in sickle cell anemia [1] and diabetes mellitus [37] we investigated whether RBC from patients with PV had abnormal interactions with endothelium by measuring RBC adhesion to human umbilical vein endothelial cells (HUVEC) under static and flow conditions. We observed an increase in the adhesion of RBC from patients with PV to HUVEC measured under static or flow conditions [5]. In PV, Lu/BCAM was overexpressed on RBC, and this increase was similar to that reported in sickle cell anemia [4]. Lu/BCAM are two glycoprotein isoforms, Lu and Lu(v13), of the immunoglobulin superfamily that carry both Lutheran blood group and basal cell adhesion molecule antigens. Lu/BCAM protein is the receptor for laminin $\alpha 5$ chain (present in laminin-10/11 isoforms) [64; 65; 66]. Lu/BCAM proteins have been also recognized as laminin $\alpha 5$ receptor in kidney epithelial cells, in smooth muscle cells and endothelial cell lines [67; 68]. The specific cytoplasmic domain of Lu/BCAMgp includes serine phosphorylation sites, which is consistent with a receptor signaling function.

The increased adhesion of PV RBC to HUVEC is mediated by erythroid Lu/BCAM and endothelial laminin $\alpha 5$. The inhibition of RBC adhesion by anti-Lu/BCAM antibody under flow condition was more pronounced than under static condition [5]. These data suggest existence of a high affinity adhesive interaction which could occur in the microcirculation. Laminins are major structural elements of all basal lamina, forming self assembling networks.

In addition to laminin $\alpha 5$ chain, integrin $\alpha 3\beta 1$ might be involved in the adhesive process since anti-$\alpha 3$ partially inhibited adhesion of PV RBC. Anti-$\beta 1$ did not inhibit adhesion but in HUVEC $\beta 1$ integrin can be associated with $\alpha 2$, $\alpha 5$, and $\alpha 6$ integrins as well as $\alpha 3$ integrin; Consequently a higher number of $\beta 1$ molecules is expressed (2×10^5 SABC) as compared to $\alpha 3$ (5×10^4 SABC) which may explain the difference between the anti-$\alpha 3$ and anti-$\beta 1$ inhibitory activity.

The interaction of laminin α5 chain with α3β1 and α6β1 has been shown in several cell types including endothelial cells [69].

JAK2 mutations found in patients with PV [60; 61] may be responsible not only for myeloproliferation and increased blood cell production but also for functional abnormalities. Lu/BCAM is expressed after Band 3 during erythropoiesis and it first appears on early orthochromatic erythroblasts [70]. Phosphorylations are essential steps during erythropoiesis as exemplified by JAK2 mutation, and these may amplify the adhesiveness of PV RBC. We recently showed that adhesion of erythroid cells expressing the Lu/BCAM long isoform to laminin α5 was increased after phosphorylation by PKA [4]. We observed that Lu/BCAMgp was spontaneously phosphorylated in RBC from PV patients. Activating the PKA signaling pathway did not increase phosphorylation of PV RBC Lu/BCAM in contrast to sickle RBC [71]. Lu/BCAM phosphorylation could account for the increased adhesion of PV RBC to laminin α5 expressed at the HUVEC surface in the absence of stimulation.

In experiments using K562 cells transfected either with JAK2 WT or JAK2 V617F we demonstrated that the presence of JAK2 V617F increased Lu/BCAM expression and to a larger extent Lu/BCAM phosphorylation. These results strongly suggest a relationship between JAK2 mutation and Lu/BCAM phosphorylation. However from these experiments we cannot conclude a direct link between JAK2 mutation and Lu/BCAM phosphorylation.

JAK2 signaling in the erythroid lineage is tightly linked to the erythropoietin receptor (EpoR), both proteins being extensively studied in normal and cancer tissues [72; 73]. Under physiological conditions, Epo binding to EpoR triggers the phosphorylation and activation of EpoR-bound JAK2, which in turn activates several downstream signaling pathways that include STAT5, PI3K/Akt, and ERK/MAPK [74]. Although the V617F substitution results in a constitutively active JAK2, its activation of the downstream signaling pathways inducing cell proliferation requires the presence of cytokine receptors, such as EpoR or the thrombopoietin receptor TpoR.18. Our finding that Lu/BCAM was phosphorylated in circulating PV *versus* healthy RBCs [5] strongly suggested that JAK2V617F would still be active in PV RBCs, raising the question about the triggered signaling pathway(s) in the absence of EpoR. JAK2V617F induces Lu/BCAM phosphorylation and activates its mediated cell adhesion to laminin by stimulating a Rap1/Akt signaling pathway in the absence of EpoR. We have previously found that Lu/BCAM adhesion function was increased in PV RBCs and here we characterize the signaling pathway responsible for this activation [75]. This pathway

involves JAK2V617F, Rap1 and Akt, as inhibiting one of these three proteins inhibits PV RBC adhesion to laminin. The JAK2V617F/PI3K/Akt pathway is well described in myeloproliferative neoplasms but this is the first time Rap1 is identified as a downstream effector of JAK2V617F.

One of our major findings is the persistence of an active JAK2V617F/Akt signaling pathway in mature PV RBCs despite the absence of EpoR. In HEL cells, silencing EpoR did not abrogate Lu/BCAM activation, indicating that it was independent of the well-described EpoR/JAK2/PI3K/Akt pathway [76].JAK2V617F has been extensively studied for its role in cell proliferation, survival and differentiation during erythropoiesis. Despite the constitutive activation feature of the V617F mutation, several reports showed that JAK2V617F-mediated

transformation requires a homodimeric type I cytokine receptor [77]. This receptor plays the role of a scaffold for the JAK2V617F-mediated signal transduction. Indeed, tyrosine phosphorylation of EpoR cytoplasmic domain is important for the activation of the downstream pathways involving STATs and PI3K/Akt [78; 79]. Hence, we investigated the presence of class I and class II cytokine receptor constituents such as gp130 subunit (class I) and interferon-α/β R1 (IFNAR1, class II) on PV and control RBCs. Flow cytometry analysis showed that gp130 and IFNAR1 were not expressed on either cell types

Although no report described the presence of cytokine receptors on RBCs, further experiments are needed to investigate their potential expression on the surface of PV RBCs. Nevertheless, this is not the first time JAK2 is shown to act independently of a receptor tyrosine kinase as Dawson and collaborators reported that human JAK2 was present in the nucleus of hematopoietic cells and directly phosphorylated histone H3 [80].

Rap1 was specifically activated in a JAK2V617F context as BaF3 JAK2V617F cells had 2.5-fold more Rap1-GTP than BaF3 JAK2 wt cells. Rap1 is a small GTPbound protein of the Ras superfamily that has been described as an upstream effector of Akt in several reports [81; 82; 83]. Ras-like proteins couple extracellular signals to various cellular responses and have the specificity of activating proteins at the inner surface of cell membranes. Rap1 is mainly involved in controlling cell adhesion, cell junction formation, cell secretion and cell polarity. The GDP-GTP cycle is regulated by guanine nucleotide-exchange factors (GEFs), which allow the GTP to bind to Rap1 after the GDP is released. Rap1 can be activated by several GEFs, such as C3G [84], Epac1 and Epac2 [85]. C3G is activated upon the phosphorylation of its tyrosine residue 504 after its recruitment to the membrane by the adaptor protein c-Crk [86]. C3G is phosphorylated by the combined action of JAK2 and c-Src in NIH-3T3 cells, driving the activation of Rap1 in response to cellular stimulation with growth hormone.

Our hypothesis is that Rap1 could be activated in a similar manner in PV RBCs, HEL and BaF3 JAK2V617F cells. Consistent with this hypothesis, Feller, Arai and collaborators [87; 88] showed that Rap1 was activated by C3G and a member of the Crk family, CrkL, that is predominantly expressed in hematopoietic cells and phosphorylated in response to stimulation with Epo or IL-3[89]. In their study, Arai and collaborators showed that adhesion of the 32D hematopoietic cell line was activated by Epo or IL-3 through the activation of the C3G/CrkL complex, Rap1- and β1 integrins.

Lu/BCAM adhesion function could be activated by the phosphorylation of its serine 62112 or by the dissociation of its cytoplasmic domain from the spectrin-based skeleton.[90; 91]. In sickle cell disease, RBCs exhibit an abnormal cAMP-dependent Lu/BCAM phosphorylation [4; 7] associated with high adhesion to laminin. This adhesion seems to involve protein kinase A14 or Rap1.22 Our findings indicate that Lu/BCAM activation could occur through another serine/threonine kinase, Akt (or protein kinase B). The in vitro phosphorylation experiments revealed that Akt could directly phosphorylate Lu cytoplasmic domain and this was strongly supported by our experiments in HEL cells where Akti inhibited Lu phosphorylation. Inhibiting PKA activity by PKAi or H89 did not impact HEL-Lu cell adhesion or Lu phosphorylation, clearly indicating that it was not involved in Lu activation in the presence of a JAK2V617F background. As increased Lu/BCAM phosphorylation could also result from serine phosphatase inhibition, we investigated the enzymatic activity of protein phosphatase 2 (PP2A), a ubiquitous serine/threonine phosphatase with broad substrate specificity. JAK2 was shown to bind to PP2A in 32D myeloid progenitor cells and to phosphorylate its catalytic subunit resulting in inhibition of phosphatase activity.

Thrombosis is the main clinical complication in PV. Growing evidence supports the hypothesis that endothelial dysfunction might contribute to thrombotic events by orchestrating the recruitment of blood cell elements to sites of injury. In PV patients with Budd-Chiari syndrome and portal vein thrombosis, Sozer and collaborators showed that cells with endothelial characteristics lining liver sinusoids and venules were JAK2V617F positive [92]. Using an immunodeficient mouse transplant assay system, the same group showed that JAK2V617F positive CD34+ cells were able to generate endothelial like cells *in vivo* expressing human JAK2V617F. Endothelial cells express a wide range of adhesion proteins including integrins and CAMs (Cell Adhesion Molecules). We show that JAK2V617F is able to activate Lu/BCAM through Rap1 and Akt that are both ubiquitously expressed proteins regulating cell adhesion and cell-cell interactions. Hence, it would be challenging to test the adhesive properties of endothelial cells expressing JAK2V617F and their recruitment potential of blood components under flow conditions.

In conclusion JAK2V617F activates an erythroid adhesion protein through a novel EpoR-independent pathway. Considering the ubiquitous feature of this signaling pathway, we assume that this activation could occur in most cell types expressing JAK2V617F and could affect other adhesion proteins than Lu/BCAM. Our work opens new perspectives in understanding cell adhesion and cell-cell interactions in human pathologies characterized by the JAK2V617F mutation.

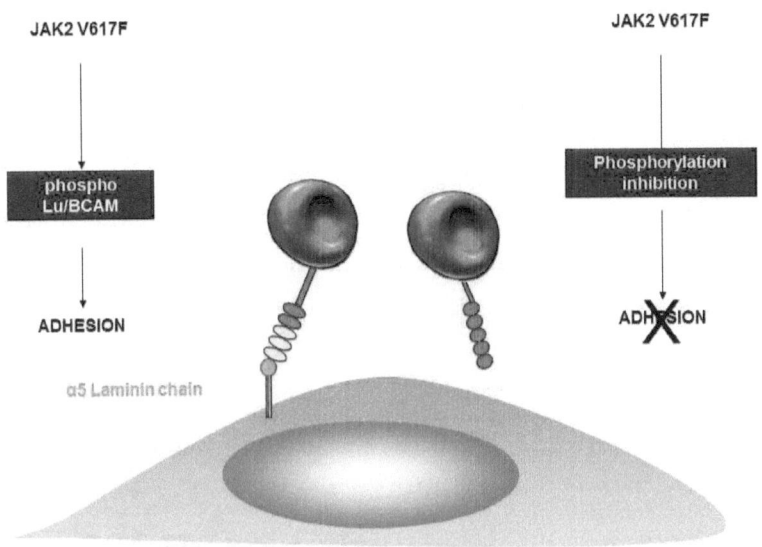

Polycythemia Vera (PV)

The increased adhesion of PV RBC to HUVEC is mediated by erythroid Lu/BCAM and endothelial laminin α5. Lu/BCAM was spontaneously phosphorylated in RBC from PV patients. Lu/BCAM phosphorylation could account for the increased adhesion of PV RBC to laminin α5 expressed at the HUVEC surface in the absence of stimulation.

Retinal Vein Occlusion

Retinal vein occlusion (RVO) is a common cause of permanent visual loss. The most frequent and less severe type, is branch retinal vein occlusion (BRVO) [93]. The most rare and sight-threatening form, central retinal vein occlusion (CRVO) remains of unknown pathophysiology [94; 95]. Aging, arterial hypertension, and glaucoma are the only well-established risk factors of RVO [96; 97; 98].

A population-based study where Retinal Branch Vein Occlusion (RBVO) and Retinal Central Vein Occlusion (RCVO) were detected at baseline (n=4,068 participants 43-86 years of age, 1988-90) and three 5-year follow-up examinations by grading 30 E color fundus photographs using standardized protocols. The prevalence of RBVO and RCVO were 0.6 and 0.1%, respectively. Using a generalized estimating equation model, while controlling for age and sex, prevalent RBVO was related to systolic blood pressure (odds ratio [OR] per 10 mmHg, 1.70, 95% confidence interval [CI] 1.13,1.50, diastolic blood pressure (OR 1.68, 95% CI 1.23,2.30), diabetes mellitus (OR 2.43, 95% CI 1.04,5.70), hypertension (OR 5.42, 95% CI 2.18,13.47), and ocular perfusion pressure (OR per 10mmHg, 2.09, 95% CI 1.45,3.02). The 15-year cumulative incidence of RBVO and RCVO was 1.8% and 0.5%, respectively. The incidence was similar in men and women and rose with age. Using a generalized estimating equation model, while controlling for age and sex, incident RBVO was related to smoking status, (OR current vs never 1.92, 95% CI 1.00, 3.70), 5-year increase in systolic blood pressure (OR per 10 mmHg, 1.20, 95% CI 1.00,

1.45), presence of glaucoma (OR 2.53, 95% CI 1.03,6.21), focal retinal arteriolar narrowing (OR 2.74 95% CI 1.40,5.73), high serum creatinine (OR ≥1.4 vs. <1.4 mg/dL 1.88, 95% CI 1.13, 3.12), migraine headache history (OR 2.00, 95% CI 1.13, 6.57),history of barbiturate use (OR 4.12, 95% CI 1.46, 11.6), and history of chloroquine use (OR 3.62, 95% CI 1.09, 12.0). Incident RBVO was more likely to occur supero-temporally and least likely nasally. Incident RBVO resulted in a drop in visual acuity by a mean of 12 letters read correctly (53 before to 41letters after) and a 28% incidence of macular edema and a 5% incidence of proliferative retinopathy while incident RCVO resulted in a drop in visual acuity by a mean of 22 letters read correctly (54 before to 32 letters after) and was associated with a 39% incidence of macular edema and a 17% incidence of proliferative retinopathy. Combining data from the Beaver Dam Eye Study and Blue Mountains Eye Study, showed that while controlling for other risk factors Retinal Vein Occlusion (RVO) at baseline was associated with a 2 ½ increase in hazard ratio for ischemic heart disease death in those younger than 70 yr of age at baseline [99]

The haemodynamics of the retinal circulation are poorly understood. The demands on this circulation are unique because of the need to pass from a high pressure environment of the eye to a low pressure one in the orbit. This makes the control of blood flow in the low pressure venous system problematic and may result in the increased risk of venous occlusion in the retina. One way to regulate the blood flow in the vein would be with the presence of a narrowing ("throttle") in the vein as it passes out of the eye i.e. at the lamina cribrosa. This has been discovered in a few histopathological specimens but never before demonstrated *in vivo*. Using Doppler ultrasound some interesting characteristics of the circulation have been seen such as pulsatile flow in the CRV. Doppler imaging was used to detect an increase in blood velocity in the CRV at the site of the lamina cribrosa by a factor of 4. In an end artery system such as the retinal circulation this suggests that the caliber of the vein is narrower at this site. Thus reducing the blood velocity (kinetic energy) in the blood of the vein as it enters a low pressure environment according to Bernoulli's equation. The venous velocities can be particularly high at the lamina cribrosa perhaps exposing the endothelium to arterial levels of shear stress. This "throttle" was further investigated in central retinal vein occlusion before and after the intervention of radial optic neurotomy [94].

Despite a number of studies, thrombophilic risk factors have not been strongly associated with RVO, which suggests a very limited role of coagulation or anticoagulation factors in the pathophysiology of the disease [100]. Little is certain about the causes of retinal vein thrombosis. There are, however, some observations that might provide approaches to identifying contributors to thrombosis in the retinal vein. One important consideration is that the vascular endothelium plays a dominant role in limiting thrombotic responses to challenge. These mechanisms include the presence on the endothelium of components of the three major natural anticoagulant mechanisms: thrombomodulin and Endothelial Protein C Receptor (EPCR) responsible for regulating protein C activation; heparin proteoglycan responsible for stimulating the activity of antithrombin; and tissue factor pathway inhibitor, a major player in the inhibition of coagulation initiation. It is known, however, that the concentrations of these proteins on the endothelium vary greatly among different vascular beds and organs. For instance, thrombomodulin is high in the lung, moderate in the liver sinusoids and low in the brain. Furthermore, there are major differences in the regulation of the gene expression of these proteins among organs. For instance, endotoxin dramatically down regulates thrombomodulin expression in the lung while slightly up regulating gene expression in the kidney. In addition to regulation of gene expression, many of these proteins are susceptible to proteolytic or oxidant injury. This in turn may vary among vessels. Complicating these issues further is the observation that dominant causes of venous and arterial thrombosis differ. In the arterial bed, platelets are a dominant contributor to thrombosis whereas in the venous circulation changes in plasma factors dominate. The retinal vein lies in between the normal vein-artery distinction, being higher flow and pressure than the standard vein but not fulfilling the normal properties of an artery [101].

Substantial data exist suggesting that blood hyperviscosity is an important risk factor. Several blood viscosity parameters have been shown to be increased in RVO patients compared to normal subjects, including a higher hematocrit, higher whole blood viscosity, reduced red cell deformability, and enhanced index of erythrocyte aggregation [102; 103; 104; 105]. It was recently reported that about 27% of patients with CRVO exhibit spontaneous *in vitro* growth of erythroid precursors in the absence of any detectable myeloproliferative disorder [106]. Red blood cells (RBC) from patients with polycythemia vera have an abnormal CD239 (Lu/BCAM) phosphorylation, which is responsible for abnormal interactions with endothelial cells. It was previously demonstrated that abnormal erythrocyte adhesion correlated with retinopathy in diabetes mellitus [55] and with vascular occlusion in sickle cell anemia. These results prompted us to study RBC adhesion to endothelial cells in CRVO.

We demonstrated that RBC adhesion to endothelial cells was significantly increased in CRVO patients compared to normal subjects. The percentage of phosphatidyl serine (PS) positive RBC was significantly higher in CRVO patients and was correlated to RBC adhesion extent. The anti-PS receptor antibodies inhibited 55% of RBC adhesion in static conditions and about 60% in flow conditions. Annexin V, which binds to PS, was the most efficient RBC adhesion blocker in flow conditions (68 to 74 %). These results reinforce the hypothesis that PS exposure on CRVO RBC is an important parameter for the increased RBC adhesion [107] .In different diseases RBC adhesion was shown to be a factor responsible for vascular occlusion. Increased exposure of PS was observed in patients with sickle cell disease (SCD) [108] to a similar extent to that we found in CRVO (2.86±2% versus 1.8±0.1%) and vascular occlusion was only observed in certain circumstances. The percentage of CRVO RBC which adheres is small and corresponds to 76,000 RBC/mm^3, which may modify vascular functions. In a rare disease, hereditary hydrocytosis, it was reported that two patients had increased RBC adhesion to endothelial cells as well as membrane phospholipid asymmetry and the authors suggested that the increased adhesion may be related to PS exposure [109]. Phospholipid asymmetry is regulated by an ATP-dependent aminophospholipid translocase (APLT) [110; 111]. Asymmetry may be lost by activation of the phospholipid scramblase (PLSCR), which causes non-specific bidirectional transport of phospholipids across the RBC membrane [112]. It has been postulated that both inhibition of APLT and activation of PLSCR result in PS externalization. Externalization of erythrocyte PS occurs in SCD [113] and may be important in the pathophysiology of vascular dysfunction in SCD and also in CRVO. The observation that RBC PS exposure is increased in patients with CRVO may represent a risk factor that can be easily explored in patients with retinal vascular occlusion.

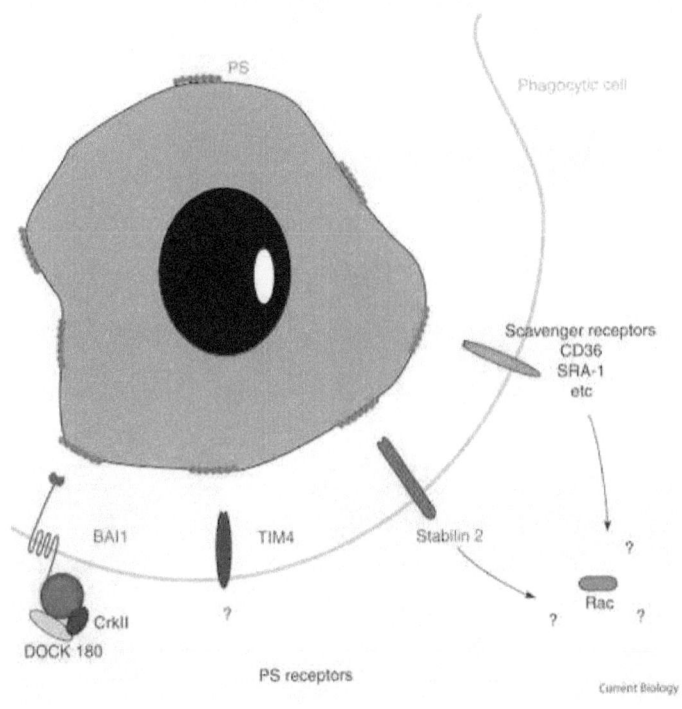

Phosphatidylserine (PS) receptors

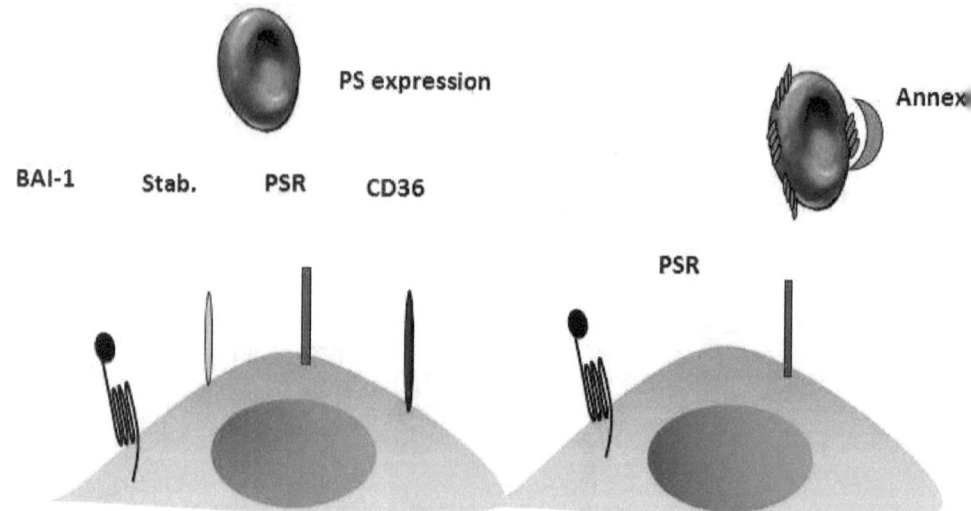

Retinal Vein Occlusion

RBCs from patients with Retinal Vein Occlusion have an enhanced PS expression and adhere to endothelium. Antibodies directed against potential PS receptors including Brain-specific Angiogenesis inhibitor (BAI-1), Stabilin-2, a scavenger receptor (stab), Phosphatidylserine receptor (PSR), and CD36, a scavenger receptor, demonstrated that the most efficient adhesion blocker was anti-PS receptor. Annexin V, which binds to PS, was the most efficient RBC adhesion blocker in flow conditions

Conclusion

Different RBC molecules and different endothelial cell receptors have been identified to be responsible for the abnormal RBC-Endothelium interactions.

In Malaria the red blood cell interaction with endothelium is complex, variable depending on the location of the endothelium. Inter Cellular Adhesion Molecule (ICAM-1) appears as a ligand for *Plasmodium falciparum* erythrocyte membrane protein1 (PfEMP1). CD36 present on the endothelium could be involved in the adhesion of red blood cells infected by the parasite. Other structures such as endothelial CD31, Platelet Endothelial Cell Adhesion Molecule-1 (PECAM-1) and glycosaminoglycans also bind to PfEMP1. In Diabetes Mellitus RBC Band 3 protein is glycated and binds to the receptor for Advanced Glycation End Products (RAGE). In PV the mutation of the kinase JAK2 results in phosphorylation of LuBCAM (CD239) which is a ligand for endothelial laminin alpha5 chain. The same RBC molecule CD239 is implicated in RBC adhesion in SCD.

These different examples indicated that RBC adhesion to endothelium may participate in the development of vascular complications in several diseases through different adhesion mechanisms. In SCD and PV a relationship between abnormal erythropoiesis and abnormal RBC behaviour has been proposed. Further studies are needed to investigate the link between bone marrow progenitor cells and mature red cell abnormalities in CRVO disease.

In SCD, treatment by hydroxyurea reduced RBC adhesion. Hydroxyurea is also the first line treatment of PV patients reducing the risk of thrombotic events. We can expect that in various diseases with increased RBC adhesion treatment correcting the RBC abnormalities or modifying adhesion molecules expression may improve the risk of vascular complications.

Modulation of ATP-dependent aminophospholipid translocase (APLT) and phospholipid scramblase (PLSCR), which regulate phospholipid asymmetry, are possible candidates for the treatment of patients with CRVO, as are the potential uses of annexin V or annexin peptides for masking PS at achievable concentrations.

References

[1] R.P. Hebbel, M.A. Boogaerts, J.W. Eaton, M.H. Steinberg, Erythrocyte adherence to endothelium in sickle-cell anemia. A possible determinant of disease severity. N Engl J Med 302 (1980) 992-995.

[2] J.L. Wautier, F. Galacteros, M.P. Wautier, D. Pintigny, Y. Beuzard, J. Rosa, J.P. Caen, Clinical manifestations and erythrocyte adhesion to endothelium in sickle cell syndrome. Am J Hematol 19 (1985) 121-130.

[3] J.L. Wautier, D. Pintigny, M.P. Wautier, R.C. Paton, F. Galacteros, P. Passa, J.P. Caen, Fibrinogen, a modulator of erythrocyte adhesion to vascular endothelium. J Lab Clin Med 101 (1983) 911-920.

[4] E. Gauthier, C. Rahuel, M.P. Wautier, W. El Nemer, P. Gane, J.L. Wautier, J.P. Cartron, Y. Colin, C. Le Van Kim, Protein kinase A-dependent phosphorylation of Lutheran/basal cell adhesion molecule glycoprotein regulates cell adhesion to laminin alpha5. J Biol Chem 280 (2005) 30055-30062.

[5] M.P. Wautier, W. El Nemer, P. Gane, J.D. Rain, J.P. Cartron, Y. Colin, C. Le Van Kim, J.L. Wautier, Increased adhesion to endothelial cells of erythrocytes from patients with polycythemia vera is mediated by laminin alpha5 chain and Lu/BCAM. Blood 110 (2007) 894-901.

[6] W. El Nemer, M.P. Wautier, C. Rahuel, P. Gane, P. Hermand, F. Galacteros, J.L. Wautier, J.P. Cartron, Y. Colin, C. Le Van Kim, Endothelial Lu/BCAM glycoproteins are novel ligands for red blood cell alpha4beta1 integrin: role in adhesion of sickle red blood cells to endothelial cells. Blood 109 (2007) 3544-3551.

[7] K. Sugihara, T. Sugihara, N. Mohandas, R.P. Hebbel, Thrombospondin mediates adherence of CD36+ sickle reticulocytes to endothelial cells. Blood 80 (1992) 2634-2642.

[8] K. Lee, P. Gane, F. Roudot-Thoraval, B. Godeau, D. Bachir, F. Bernaudin, J.P. Cartron, F. Galacteros, P. Bierling, The nonexpression of CD36 on reticulocytes and mature red blood cells does not modify the clinical course of patients with sickle cell anemia. Blood 98 (2001) 966-971.

[9] P. Hermand, P. Gane, I. Callebaut, N. Kieffer, J.P. Cartron, P. Bailly, Integrin receptor specificity for human red cell ICAM-4 ligand. Critical residues for alphaIIbeta3 binding. Eur J Biochem 271 (2004) 3729-3740.

[10] S. Charache, M.L. Terrin, R.D. Moore, G.J. Dover, F.B. Barton, S.V. Eckert, R.P. McMahon, D.R. Bonds, Effect of hydroxyurea on the frequency of painful crises in sickle cell anemia. Investigators of the Multicenter Study of Hydroxyurea in Sickle Cell Anemia. N Engl J Med 332 (1995) 1317-1322.

[11] D.K. Kaul, X.D. Liu, X. Zhang, T. Mankelow, S. Parsons, F. Spring, X. An, N. Mohandas, D. Anstee, J.A. Chasis, Peptides based on alphaV-binding domains of erythrocyte ICAM-4 inhibit sickle red cell-endothelial interactions and vaso-occlusion in the microcirculation. Am J Physiol Cell Physiol 291 (2006) C922-930.

[12] P. Bartolucci, V. Chaar, J. Picot, D. Bachir, A. Habibi, C. Fauroux, F. Galacteros, Y. Colin, C. Le Van Kim, W. El Nemer, Decreased sickle red blood cell adhesion to laminin by hydroxyurea is associated with inhibition of Lu/BCAM protein phosphorylation. Blood 116 (2010) 2152-2159.

[13] S. Lecourt, V. Vanneaux, A. Cras, D. Freida, D. Heraoui, L. Herbi, C. Caillaud, C. Chomienne, J.P. Marolleau, N. Belmatoug, J. Larghero, Bone marrow microenvironment in an in vitro model of Gaucher disease: consequences of glucocerebrosidase deficiency. Stem cells and development 21 (2012) 239-248.

[14] P.K. Mistry, J. Liu, M. Yang, T. Nottoli, J. McGrath, D. Jain, K. Zhang, J. Keutzer, W.L. Chuang, W.Z. Mehal, H. Zhao, A. Lin, S. Mane, X. Liu, Y.Z. Peng, J.H. Li, M. Agrawal, L.L. Zhu, H.C. Blair, L.J. Robinson, J. Iqbal, L. Sun, M. Zaidi, Glucocerebrosidase gene-deficient mouse recapitulates Gaucher disease displaying cellular and molecular dysregulation beyond the macrophage. Proc Natl Acad Sci U S A 107 (2010) 19473-19478.

[15] J. Berger, S. Lecourt, V. Vanneaux, C. Rapatel, S. Boisgard, C. Caillaud, N. Boiret-Dupre, C. Chomienne, J.P. Marolleau, J. Larghero, M.G. Berger,

Glucocerebrosidase deficiency dramatically impairs human bone marrow haematopoiesis in an in vitro model of Gaucher disease. Br J Haematol 150 (2010) 93-101.

[16] M. Franco, E. Collec, P. Connes, E. van den Akker, T. Billette de Villemeur, N. Belmatoug, M. von Lindern, N. Ameziane, O. Hermine, Y. Colin, C. Le Van Kim, C. Mignot, Abnormal properties of red blood cells suggest a role in the pathophysiology of Gaucher disease. Blood 121 (2013) 546-555.

[17] A.G. Maier, B.M. Cooke, A.F. Cowman, L. Tilley, Malaria parasite proteins that remodel the host erythrocyte. Nat Rev Microbiol 7 (2009) 341-354.

[18] P. Lim, C. Wongsrichanalai, P. Chim, N. Khim, S. Kim, S. Chy, R. Sem, S. Nhem, P. Yi, S. Duong, D.M. Bouth, B. Genton, H.P. Beck, J.G. Gobert, W.O. Rogers, J.Y. Coppee, T. Fandeur, O. Mercereau-Puijalon, P. Ringwald, J. Le Bras, F. Ariey, Decreased in vitro susceptibility of Plasmodium falciparum isolates to artesunate, mefloquine, chloroquine, and quinine in Cambodia from 2001 to 2007. Antimicrob Agents Chemother 54 2135-2142.

[19] L.H. Miller, M.F. Good, G. Milon, Malaria pathogenesis. Science 264 (1994) 1878-1883.

[20] T. Lavstsen, A. Salanti, A.T. Jensen, D.E. Arnot, T.G. Theander, Sub-grouping of Plasmodium falciparum 3D7 var genes based on sequence analysis of coding and non-coding regions. Malar J 2 (2003) 27.

[21] K.R. Hughes, G.A. Biagini, A.G. Craig, Continued cytoadherence of Plasmodium falciparum infected red blood cells after antimalarial treatment. Mol Biochem Parasitol (2010) 169 71-78.

[22] B.A. Robinson, T.L. Welch, J.D. Smith, Widespread functional specialization of Plasmodium falciparum erythrocyte membrane protein 1 family members to bind CD36 analysed across a parasite genome. Mol Microbiol 47 (2003) 1265-1278.

[23] Q. Chen, A. Heddini, A. Barragan, V. Fernandez, S.F. Pearce, M. Wahlgren, The semiconserved head structure of Plasmodium falciparum erythrocyte membrane protein 1 mediates binding to multiple independent host receptors. J Exp Med 192 (2000) 1-10.

[24] C.J. Treutiger, A. Heddini, V. Fernandez, W.A. Muller, M. Wahlgren, PECAM-1/CD31, an endothelial receptor for binding Plasmodium falciparum-infected erythrocytes. Nat Med 3 (1997) 1405-1408.

[25] K.L. Waller, L.M. Stubberfield, V. Dubljevic, D.W. Buckingham, N. Mohandas, R.L. Coppel, B.M. Cooke, Interaction of the exported malaria protein Pf332 with the red blood cell membrane skeleton. Biochimica et biophysica acta 1798 (2010) 861-871.

[26] M.C. Nunes, M. Okada, C. Scheidig-Benatar, B.M. Cooke, A. Scherf, Plasmodium falciparum FIKK kinase members target distinct components of the erythrocyte membrane. PloS one 5 (2010) e11747.

[27] L. Joergensen, D.C. Bengtsson, A. Bengtsson, E. Ronander, S.S. Berger, L. Turner, M.B. Dalgaard, G.K. Cham, M.E. Victor, T. Lavstsen, T.G. Theander, D.E. Arnot, A.T. Jensen, Surface co-expression of two different PfEMP1 antigens on single plasmodium falciparum-infected erythrocytes facilitates binding to ICAM1 and PECAM1. PLoS Pathog 6 e1001083.

[28] A. Officers, A.C.R.G.T.A. Coordinators for the, T. Lipid-Lowering Treatment to Prevent Heart Attack, Major outcomes in high-risk hypertensive patients randomized to angiotensin-converting enzyme inhibitor or calcium channel blocker vs diuretic: The Antihypertensive and Lipid-Lowering Treatment to Prevent Heart Attack Trial (ALLHAT). JAMA : the journal of the American Medical Association 288 (2002) 2981-2997.

[29] B. Dahlof, P.S. Sever, N.R. Poulter, H. Wedel, D.G. Beevers, M. Caulfield, R. Collins, S.E. Kjeldsen, A. Kristinsson, G.T. McInnes, J. Mehlsen, M. Nieminen, E. O'Brien, J. Ostergren, A. Investigators, Prevention of cardiovascular events with an antihypertensive regimen of amlodipine adding perindopril as required versus atenolol adding bendroflumethiazide as required, in the Anglo-Scandinavian Cardiac Outcomes Trial-Blood Pressure Lowering Arm (ASCOT-BPLA): a multicentre randomised controlled trial. Lancet 366 (2005) 895-906.

[30] S.M. Marshall, A. Flyvbjerg, Prevention and early detection of vascular complications of diabetes. Bmj 333 (2006) 475-480.

[31] Tight blood pressure control and risk of macrovascular and microvascular complications in type 2 diabetes: UKPDS 38. UK Prospective Diabetes Study Group. Bmj 317 (1998) 703-713.

[32] E.L. Bierman, George Lyman Duff Memorial Lecture. Atherogenesis in diabetes. Arteriosclerosis and thrombosis : a journal of vascular biology / American Heart Association 12 (1992) 647-656.

[33] W.B. Kannel, D.L. McGee, Diabetes and cardiovascular disease. The Framingham study. JAMA : the journal of the American Medical Association 241 (1979) 2035-2038.

[34] G.L. King, M. Brownlee, The cellular and molecular mechanisms of diabetic complications. Endocrinology and metabolism clinics of North America 25 (1996) 255-270.

[35] A.S. Krolewski, E.J. Kosinski, J.H. Warram, O.S. Leland, E.J. Busick, A.C. Asmal, L.I. Rand, A.R. Christlieb, R.F. Bradley, C.R. Kahn, Magnitude and determinants of coronary artery disease in juvenile-onset, insulin-dependent diabetes mellitus. The American journal of cardiology 59 (1987) 750-755.

[36] A.M. Schmidt, S.D. Yan, J.L. Wautier, D. Stern, Activation of receptor for advanced glycation end products: a mechanism for chronic vascular dysfunction in diabetic vasculopathy and atherosclerosis. Circ Res 84 (1999) 489-497.

[37] J.L. Wautier, R.C. Paton, M.P. Wautier, D. Pintigny, E. Abadie, P. Passa, J.P. Caen, Increased adhesion of erythrocytes to endothelial cells in diabetes mellitus and its relation to vascular complications. N Engl J Med 305 (1981) 237-242.

[38] J.L. Wautier, H. LeBlanc, M.P. Wautier, E. Abadie, P. Passa, J.P. Caen, Erythrocyte adhesion to cultured endothelium and glycaemic control in type 1 (insulin-dependent) diabetic patients. Diabetologia 29 (1986) 151-155.

[39] J.L. Wautier, M.P. Wautier, A.M. Schmidt, G.M. Anderson, O. Hori, C. Zoukourian, L. Capron, O. Chappey, S.D. Yan, J. Brett, et al., Advanced glycation end products (AGEs) on the surface of diabetic erythrocytes bind to the vessel wall via a specific receptor inducing oxidant stress in the vasculature: a link between surface-associated AGEs and diabetic complications. Proc Natl Acad Sci U S A 91 (1994) 7742-7746.

[40] C. Zoukourian, M.P. Wautier, O. Chappey, C. Dosquet, T. Rohban, A.M. Schmidt, D. Stern, J.L. Wautier, Endothelial cell dysfunction secondary to the adhesion of diabetic erythrocytes. Modulation by iloprost.

International angiology : a journal of the International Union of Angiology 15 (1996) 195-200.

[41] Wautier JL, Schmidt AM, Protein glycation: a firm link to endothelial cell dysfunction. Circ Res 95 (2004) 233-238.

[42] Wautier MP, Chappey O, Corda S, Stern DM, Schmidt AM, Wautier JL, Activation of NADPH oxidase by AGE links oxidant stress to altered gene expression via RAGE. Am. J. Physiol. Endocrinol. Metab. 280 (2001) E685-694.

[43] Wautier JL, Zoukourian C, Chappey O, Wautier MP, Guillausseau PJ, Cao R, Hori O, Stern D, Schmidt AM, Receptor-mediated endothelial cell dysfunction in diabetic vasculopathy. Soluble receptor for advanced glycation end products blocks hyperpermeability in diabetic rats. J Clin Invest 97 (1996) 238-243.

[44] Renard C, Chappey O, Wautier MP, Nagashima M, Morser J, Scherrmann JM, Wautier JL, The human and rat recombinant receptors for advanced glycation end products have a high degree of homology but different pharmacokinetic properties in rats. J Pharmacol Exp Ther 290 (1999) 1458-1466.

[45] Zoukourian C, Wautier MP, Chappey O, Dosquet C, Rohban T, Schmidt AM, Stern D, Wautier JL, Endothelial cell dysfunction secondary to the adhesion of diabetic erythrocytes. Modulation by iloprost. Int Angiol 15 (1996) 195-200.

[46] Wautier MP, Massin P, Guillausseau PJ, Huijberts M, Levy B, Boulanger E, Laloi-Michelin M, Wautier JL, N(carboxymethyl)lysine as a biomarker for microvascular complications in type 2 diabetic patients. Diabetes Metab. 29 (2003) 44-52.

[47] Wautier MP, Khodabandehlou T, Le Devehat C, Wautier JL, Modulation of RAGE expression influences the adhesion of red blood cells from diabetic patients. Clin. Hemorheol. Microcirc. 35 (2006) 379-386.

[48] Zhan CD, Sindhu RK, Vaziri ND, Up-regulation of kidney NAD(P)H oxidase and calcineurin in SHR: reversal by lifelong antioxidant supplementation. Kidney Int 65 (2004) 219-227.

[49] Gorlach A, Brandes RP, Nguyen K, Amidi M, Dehghani F, Busse R, A gp91phox containing NADPH oxidase selectively expressed in

endothelial cells is a major source of oxygen radical generation in the arterial wall. Circ Res 87 (2000) 26-32.

[50] Wassmann S, Wassmann K, Nickenig G, Modulation of oxidant and antioxidant enzyme expression and function in vascular cells. Hypertension 44 (2004) 381-386.

[51] Toth J, Racz A, Kaminski PM, Wolin MS, Bagi Z, Koller A, Asymmetrical dimethylarginine inhibits shear stress-induced nitric oxide release and dilation and elicits superoxide-mediated increase in arteriolar tone. Hypertension 49 (2007) 563-568.

[52] Marx N, Walcher D, Ivanova N, Rautzenberg K, Jung A, Friedl R, Hombach V, de Caterina R, Basta G, Wautier MP, Wautier JL, Thiazolidinediones reduce endothelial expression of receptors for advanced glycation end products. Diabetes 53 (2004) 2662-2668.

[53] Park L, Raman KG, Lee KJ, Lu Y, Ferran LJ Jr, Chow WS, Stern D, Schmidt AM, Suppression of accelerated diabetic atherosclerosis by the soluble receptor for advanced glycation endproducts. Nat Med 4 (1998) 1025-1031.

[54] N. Grossin, M.P. Wautier, J. Picot, D.M. Stern, J.L. Wautier, Differential effect of plasma or erythrocyte AGE-ligands of RAGE on expression of transcripts for receptor isoforms. Diabetes Metab 35 (2009) 410-417.

[55] M.P. Wautier, E. Boulanger, P.J. Guillausseau, P. Massin, J.L. Wautier, AGEs, macrophage colony stimulating factor and vascular adhesion molecule blood levels are increased in patients with diabetic microangiopathy. Thromb Haemost 91 (2004) 879-885.

[56] R. Tamarat, J.S. Silvestre, M. Huijberts, J. Benessiano, T.G. Ebrahimian, M. Duriez, M.P. Wautier, J.L. Wautier, B.I. Levy, Blockade of advanced glycation end-product formation restores ischemia-induced angiogenesis in diabetic mice. Proc Natl Acad Sci U S A 100 (2003) 8555-8560.

[57] M.P. Wautier, T. Khodabandehlou, C. Le Devehat, J.L. Wautier, Modulation of RAGE expression influences the adhesion of red blood cells from diabetic patients. Clin Hemorheol Microcirc 35 (2006) 379-386.

[58] J.L. Wautier, A.M. Schmidt, Protein glycation: a firm link to endothelial cell dysfunction. Circ Res 95 (2004) 233-238.

[59] J.T. Prchal, Polycythemia vera and other primary polycythemias. Curr Opin Hematol 12 (2005) 112-116.

[60] E.J. Baxter, L.M. Scott, P.J. Campbell, C. East, N. Fourouclas, S. Swanton, G.S. Vassiliou, A.J. Bench, E.M. Boyd, N. Curtin, M.A. Scott, W.N. Erber, A.R. Green, Acquired mutation of the tyrosine kinase JAK2 in human myeloproliferative disorders. Lancet 365 (2005) 1054-1061.

[61] C. James, V. Ugo, J.P. Le Couedic, J. Staerk, F. Delhommeau, C. Lacout, L. Garcon, H. Raslova, R. Berger, A. Bennaceur-Griscelli, J.L. Villeval, S.N. Constantinescu, N. Casadevall, W. Vainchenker, A unique clonal JAK2 mutation leading to constitutive signalling causes polycythaemia vera. Nature 434 (2005) 1144-1148.

[62] L.M. Scott, W. Tong, R.L. Levine, M.A. Scott, P.A. Beer, M.R. Stratton, P.A. Futreal, W.N. Erber, M.F. McMullin, C.N. Harrison, A.J. Warren, D.G. Gilliland, H.F. Lodish, A.R. Green, JAK2 exon 12 mutations in polycythemia vera and idiopathic erythrocytosis. N Engl J Med 356 (2007) 459-468.

[63] V. De Stefano, A. Fiorini, E. Rossi, T. Za, G. Farina, P. Chiusolo, S. Sica, G. Leone, Incidence of the JAK2 V617F mutation among patients with splanchnic or cerebral venous thrombosis and without overt chronic myeloproliferative disorders. J Thromb Haemost 5 (2007) 708-714.

[64] W. El Nemer, P. Gane, Y. Colin, V. Bony, C. Rahuel, F. Galacteros, J.P. Cartron, C. Le Van Kim, The Lutheran blood group glycoproteins, the erythroid receptors for laminin, are adhesion molecules. J Biol Chem 273 (1998) 16686-16693.

[65] M. Udani, Q. Zen, M. Cottman, N. Leonard, S. Jefferson, C. Daymont, G. Truskey, M.J. Telen, Basal cell adhesion molecule/lutheran protein. The receptor critical for sickle cell adhesion to laminin. J Clin Invest 101 (1998) 2550-2558.

[66] S.F. Parsons, G. Lee, F.A. Spring, T.N. Willig, L.L. Peters, J.A. Gimm, M.J. Tanner, N. Mohandas, D.J. Anstee, J.A. Chasis, Lutheran blood group glycoprotein and its newly characterized mouse homologue specifically bind alpha5 chain-containing human laminin with high affinity. Blood 97 (2001) 312-320.

[67] A.L. Bolcato-Bellemin, O. Lefebvre, C. Arnold, L. Sorokin, J.H. Miner, M. Kedinger, P. Simon-Assmann, Laminin alpha5 chain is required for intestinal smooth muscle development. Dev Biol 260 (2003) 376-390.

[68] N. Vainionpaa, Y. Kikkawa, K. Lounatmaa, J.H. Miner, P. Rousselle, I. Virtanen, Laminin-10 and Lutheran blood group glycoproteins in adhesion of human endothelial cells. Am J Physiol Cell Physiol 290 (2006) C764-775.

[69] R. Hallmann, N. Horn, M. Selg, O. Wendler, F. Pausch, L.M. Sorokin, Expression and function of laminins in the embryonic and mature vasculature. Physiol Rev 85 (2005) 979-1000.

[70] M.J. Southcott, M.J. Tanner, D.J. Anstee, The expression of human blood group antigens during erythropoiesis in a cell culture system. Blood 93 (1999) 4425-4435.

[71] P.C. Hines, Q. Zen, S.N. Burney, D.A. Shea, K.I. Ataga, E.P. Orringer, M.J. Telen, L.V. Parise, Novel epinephrine and cyclic AMP-mediated activation of BCAM/Lu-dependent sickle (SS) RBC adhesion. Blood 101 (2003) 3281-3287.

[72] W. Jelkmann, J. Bohlius, M. Hallek, A.J. Sytkowski, The erythropoietin receptor in normal and cancer tissues. Critical reviews in oncology/hematology 67 (2008) 39-61.

[73] W. Vainchenker, A. Dusa, S.N. Constantinescu, JAKs in pathology: role of Janus kinases in hematopoietic malignancies and immunodeficiencies. Seminars in cell & developmental biology 19 (2008) 385-393.

[74] F. Delhommeau, D.F. Pisani, C. James, N. Casadevall, S. Constantinescu, W. Vainchenker, Oncogenic mechanisms in myeloproliferative disorders. Cell Mol Life Sci 63 (2006) 2939-2953.

[75] M. De Grandis, M. Cambot, M.P. Wautier, B. Cassinat, C. Chomienne, Y. Colin, J.L. Wautier, C. Le Van Kim, W. El Nemer, JAK2V617F activates Lu/BCAM-mediated red cell adhesion in polycythemia vera through an EpoR-independent Rap1/Akt pathway. Blood 121 (2013) 658-665.

[76] P.A. Tilbrook, S.P. Klinken, The erythropoietin receptor. The international journal of biochemistry & cell biology 31 (1999) 1001-1005.

[77] X. Lu, R. Levine, W. Tong, G. Wernig, Y. Pikman, S. Zarnegar, D.G. Gilliland, H. Lodish, Expression of a homodimeric type I cytokine receptor is required for JAK2V617F-mediated transformation. Proc Natl Acad Sci U S A 102 (2005) 18962-18967.

[78] J. Kamishimoto, K. Tago, T. Kasahara, M. Funakoshi-Tago, Akt activation through the phosphorylation of erythropoietin receptor at tyrosine 479 is required for myeloproliferative disorder-associated JAK2 V617F mutant-induced cellular transformation. Cellular signalling 23 (2011) 849-856.

[79] T. Kisseleva, S. Bhattacharya, J. Braunstein, C.W. Schindler, Signaling through the JAK/STAT pathway, recent advances and future challenges. Gene 285 (2002) 1-24.

[80] M.A. Dawson, A.J. Bannister, B. Gottgens, S.D. Foster, T. Bartke, A.R. Green, T. Kouzarides, JAK2 phosphorylates histone H3Y41 and excludes HP1alpha from chromatin. Nature 461 (2009) 819-822.

[81] R. Banerjee, B.S. Henson, N. Russo, A. Tsodikov, N.J. D'Silva, Rap1 mediates galanin receptor 2-induced proliferation and survival in squamous cell carcinoma. Cellular signalling 23 (2011) 1110-1118.

[82] G. Carmona, S. Gottig, A. Orlandi, J. Scheele, T. Bauerle, M. Jugold, F. Kiessling, R. Henschler, A.M. Zeiher, S. Dimmeler, E. Chavakis, Role of the small GTPase Rap1 for integrin activity regulation in endothelial cells and angiogenesis. Blood 113 (2009) 488-497.

[83] M.W. Jang, S.P. Yun, J.H. Park, J.M. Ryu, J.H. Lee, H.J. Han, Cooperation of Epac1/Rap1/Akt and PKA in prostaglandin E(2) -induced proliferation of human umbilical cord blood derived mesenchymal stem cells: involvement of c-Myc and VEGF expression. Journal of cellular physiology 227 (2012) 3756-3767.

[84] Y. Ohba, N. Mochizuki, K. Matsuo, S. Yamashita, M. Nakaya, Y. Hashimoto, M. Hamaguchi, T. Kurata, K. Nagashima, M. Matsuda, Rap2 as a slowly responding molecular switch in the Rap1 signaling cascade. Molecular and cellular biology 20 (2000) 6074-6083.

[85] J.L. Bos, H. Rehmann, A. Wittinghofer, GEFs and GAPs: critical elements in the control of small G proteins. Cell 129 (2007) 865-877.

[86] T. Ichiba, Y. Hashimoto, M. Nakaya, Y. Kuraishi, S. Tanaka, T. Kurata, N. Mochizuki, M. Matsuda, Activation of C3G guanine nucleotide exchange

factor for Rap1 by phosphorylation of tyrosine 504. J Biol Chem 274 (1999) 14376-14381.

[87] S.M. Feller, G. Posern, J. Voss, C. Kardinal, D. Sakkab, J. Zheng, B.S. Knudsen, Physiological signals and oncogenesis mediated through Crk family adapter proteins. Journal of cellular physiology 177 (1998) 535-552.

[88] A. Arai, Y. Nosaka, E. Kanda, K. Yamamoto, N. Miyasaka, O. Miura, Rap1 is activated by erythropoietin or interleukin-3 and is involved in regulation of beta1 integrin-mediated hematopoietic cell adhesion. J Biol Chem 276 (2001) 10453-10462.

[89] H. Chin, T. Saito, A. Arai, K. Yamamoto, R. Kamiyama, N. Miyasaka, O. Miura, Erythropoietin and IL-3 induce tyrosine phosphorylation of CrkL and its association with Shc, SHP-2, and Cbl in hematopoietic cells. Biochemical and biophysical research communications 239 (1997) 412-417.

[90] E. Gauthier, W. El Nemer, M.P. Wautier, O. Renaud, G. Tchernia, J. Delaunay, C. Le Van Kim, Y. Colin, Role of the interaction between Lu/BCAM and the spectrin-based membrane skeleton in the increased adhesion of hereditary spherocytosis red cells to laminin. Br J Haematol 148 (2010) 456-465.

[91] X. An, E. Gauthier, X. Zhang, X. Guo, D.J. Anstee, N. Mohandas, J.A. Chasis, Adhesive activity of Lu glycoproteins is regulated by interaction with spectrin. Blood 112 (2008) 5212-5218.

[92] S. Sozer, M.I. Fiel, T. Schiano, M. Xu, J. Mascarenhas, R. Hoffman, The presence of JAK2V617F mutation in the liver endothelial cells of patients with Budd-Chiari syndrome. Blood 113 (2009) 5246-5249.

[93] S.L. Rogers, R.L. McIntosh, L. Lim, P. Mitchell, N. Cheung, J.W. Kowalski, H.P. Nguyen, J.J. Wang, T.Y. Wong, Natural history of branch retinal vein occlusion: an evidence-based systematic review. Ophthalmology (2010) 117 1094-1101 e1095.

[94] T.H. Williamson, Central retinal vein occlusion: what's the story? Br J Ophthalmol 81 (1997) 698-704.

[95] M. Rehak, P. Wiedemann, Retinal vein thrombosis: pathogenesis and management. J Thromb Haemost (2010) 8 1886-1894.

[96] R. Marcucci, L. Bertini, B. Giusti, T. Brunelli, S. Fedi, A.P. Cellai, D. Poli, G. Pepe, R. Abbate, D. Prisco, Thrombophilic risk factors in patients with central retinal vein occlusion. Thromb Haemost 86 (2001) 772-776.

[97] M. Yasuda, Y. Kiyohara, S. Arakawa, Y. Hata, K. Yonemoto, Y. Doi, M. Iida, T. Ishibashi, Prevalence and systemic risk factors for retinal vein occlusion in a general Japanese population: the Hisayama study. Invest Ophthalmol Vis Sci (2010) 51 3205-3209.

[98] R.D. Sperduto, R. Hiller, E. Chew, D. Seigel, N. Blair, T.C. Burton, M.D. Farber, E.S. Gragoudas, J. Haller, J.M. Seddon, L.A. Yannuzzi, Risk factors for hemiretinal vein occlusion: comparison with risk factors for central and branch retinal vein occlusion: the eye disease case-control study. Ophthalmology 105 (1998) 765-771.

[99] A.B. Fernandez, T.Y. Wong, R. Klein, D. Collins, G. Burke, M.F. Cotch, B. Klein, M.M. Sadeghi, J. Chen, Age-related macular degeneration and incident cardiovascular disease: the Multi-Ethnic Study of Atherosclerosis. Ophthalmology 119 (2012) 765-770.

[100] M.C. Janssen, M. den Heijer, J.R. Cruysberg, H. Wollersheim, S.J. Bredie, Retinal vein occlusion: a form of venous thrombosis or a complication of atherosclerosis? A meta-analysis of thrombophilic factors. Thromb Haemost 93 (2005) 1021-1026.

[101] C.T. Esmon, Protein C anticoagulant system--anti-inflammatory effects. Seminars in immunopathology 34 (2012) 127-132.

[102] A. Chabanel, A. Glacet-Bernard, F. Lelong, A. Taccoen, G. Coscas, M.M. Samama, Increased red blood cell aggregation in retinal vein occlusion. Br J Haematol 75 (1990) 127-131.

[103] O. Arend, A. Remky, F. Jung, H. Kiesewetter, M. Reim, S. Wolf, Role of rheologic factors in patients with acute central retinal vein occlusion. Ophthalmology 103 (1996) 80-86.

[104] F. Sofi, L. Mannini, R. Marcucci, P. Bolli, A. Sodi, B. Giambene, U. Menchini, G.F. Gensini, R. Abbate, D. Prisco, Role of haemorheological factors in patients with retinal vein occlusion. Thromb Haemost 98 (2007) 1215-1219.

[105]S. Yedgar, D.K. Kaul, G. Barshtein, RBC adhesion to vascular endothelial cells: more potent than RBC aggregation in inducing circulatory disorders. Microcirculation 15 (2008) 581-583.

[106]E. Heron, C. Marzac, S. Feldman-Billard, J.F. Girmens, M. Paques, R. Delarue, J.C. Piette, N. Casadevall, O. Hermine, Endogenous erythroid colony formation in patients with retinal vein occlusion. Ophthalmology 114 (2007) 2155-2161.

[107]M.P. Wautier, E. Heron, J. Picot, Y. Colin, O. Hermine, J.L. Wautier, Red blood cell phosphatidylserine exposure is responsible for increased erythrocyte adhesion to endothelium in central retinal vein occlusion. J Thromb Haemost (2011) 9 1049-1055.

[108]B.L. Wood, D.F. Gibson, J.F. Tait, Increased erythrocyte phosphatidylserine exposure in sickle cell disease: flow-cytometric measurement and clinical associations. Blood 88 (1996) 1873-1880.

[109]P.G. Gallagher, S.H. Chang, M.P. Rettig, J.E. Neely, C.A. Hillery, B.D. Smith, P.S. Low, Altered erythrocyte endothelial adherence and membrane phospholipid asymmetry in hereditary hydrocytosis. Blood 101 (2003) 4625-4627.

[110]L.A. Barber, M.B. Palascak, C.H. Joiner, R.S. Franco, Aminophospholipid translocase and phospholipid scramblase activities in sickle erythrocyte subpopulations. Br J Haematol 146 (2009) 447-455.

[111]E. Soupene, F.A. Kuypers, Identification of an erythroid ATP-dependent aminophospholipid transporter. Br J Haematol 133 (2006) 436-438.

[112]J.L. Wolfs, P. Comfurius, J.T. Rasmussen, J.F. Keuren, T. Lindhout, R.F. Zwaal, E.M. Bevers, Activated scramblase and inhibited aminophospholipid translocase cause phosphatidylserine exposure in a distinct platelet fraction. Cell Mol Life Sci 62 (2005) 1514-1525.

[113]F.A. Kuypers, J. Yuan, R.A. Lewis, L.M. Snyder, C.R. Kiefer, A. Bunyaratvej, S. Fucharoen, L. Ma, L. Styles, K. de Jong, S.L. Schrier, Membrane phospholipid asymmetry in human thalassemia. Blood 91 (1998) 3044-3051.

MoreBooks!
publishing

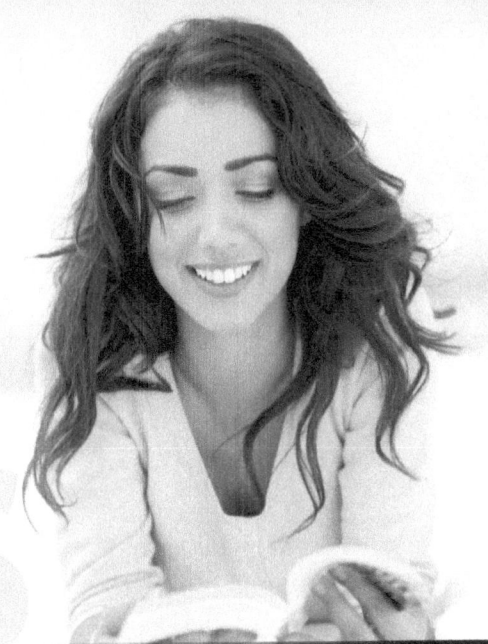

i want morebooks!

Buy your books fast and straightforward online - at one of world's fastest growing online book stores! Environmentally sound due to Print-on-Demand technologies.

Buy your books online at

www.get-morebooks.com

Kaufen Sie Ihre Bücher schnell und unkompliziert online – auf einer der am schnellsten wachsenden Buchhandelsplattformen weltweit! Dank Print-On-Demand umwelt- und ressourcenschonend produziert.

Bücher schneller online kaufen

www.morebooks.de

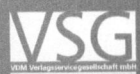

VDM Verlagsservicegesellschaft mbH
Heinrich-Böcking-Str. 6-8
D - 66121 Saarbrücken

Telefon: +49 681 3720 174
Telefax: +49 681 3720 1749

info@vdm-vsg.de
www.vdm-vsg.de

www.ingramcontent.com/pod-product-compliance
Lightning Source LLC
Chambersburg PA
CBHW031545210526
45464CB00003B/1158